THE ESSENTIAL WOMAN

Female Health and Fertility
in Chinese Classical Texts

Monkey Press is named after the Monkey King in The Journey to the West, the 16th century novel by Wu Chengen. Monkey blends skill, initiative and wisdom with the spirit of freedom, irreverence and mischief.

Also published by Monkey Press:
The Way of Heaven: Neijing Suwen chapters 1 and 2
The Secret Treatise of the Spiritual Orchid: Suwen chapter 8
The Seven Emotions
The Eight Extraordinary Meridians
The Extraordinary Fu
Essence Spirit Blood and Qi
The Lung
The Kidneys
Spleen and Stomach
The Heart in Lingshu chapter 8
The Liver
Heart Master Triple Heater
A Study of Qi
Yin Yang in Classical Texts

THE ESSENTIAL WOMAN
Female Health and Fertility
in Chinese Classical Texts

Elisabeth Rochat de la Vallée

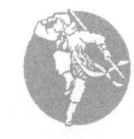

MONKEY PRESS

© Monkey Press 2007
THE ESSENTIAL WOMAN
Elisabeth Rochat de la Vallée

All rights reserved. No part of this book may be reproduced in any form without written permission from the publisher.

ISBN 978 1 872468 33 4

www.monkeypress.net
monkey.press@virgin.net

Text Editor: Caroline Root
Production and Design: Sandra Hill
Cover image: Court Women, Tang Dynasty

Printed on recycled paper by
Biddles Ltd, Kings Lynn, Norfolk

CONTENTS

BLOOD AND QI	1
Chong mai and ren mai	10
Yin and yang qiao mai	15
BAO LUO	18
Bao zhong	19
Bao luo and the kidneys	22
Uterus as extraordinary fu	23
ZANG AND FU	26
The kidneys	26
The liver	31
Spleen and stomach	38
The heart	41
The lung	45
THE EXTRAORDINARY MERIDIANS	47
Chong mai	47
Ren mai	49
Du mai	50
Dai mai	52
SUWEN CHAPTER 1	54
Seven and eight year cycles	55
Seven years old	60
Fourteen years old	61
Twenty-one years old	65
Twenty-eight years old	66

Thirty-five years old	67
Forty-two years old	69
Forty-nine years old	70
INFERTILITY	72
Emptiness of the kidneys	73
Obstruction of the liver	78
Phlegm and damp	80
Blood stasis	82
MENOPAUSE	84
Kidney yin deficiency	87
Kidney yang deficiency	90
MENSTRUAL PROBLEMS	92
Amenorrhoea	96
Dryness of the blood	96
Blood stasis	98
Liver and kidney deficiency	100
Emptiness of blood and *qi*	102
Emptiness of *yin*	104
Blockage of *qi* and blood stasis	105
Phlegm and damp	106
Invasion of heat in the blood chamber	107
Invasion by cold	118
INDEX	129

FOREWORD

What does it mean to be a woman? What are the defining qualities of the feminine? Within the philosophical and medical understanding of a cosmology dominated by the dualities of *yin yang* and blood and *qi*, one half of the male/female couple can only be understood in relation to the other. The specific nature of a woman is therefore first determined by the balance of these things, blood and *qi* and *yin* and *yang*:

> 'In the third month something is decided at the level of the balance of blood and *qi* and from then the sex of the child is determined.'

In this book Elisabeth Rochat casts a broad eye over the essential nature of a woman, drawing on a range of Chinese texts both well-known and more obscure. Starting with the balance of blood and *qi* she moves on to examine the nature of the *bao luo* (protecting envelope and uterus) and the different roles played by the *zang fu* and extraordinary meridians in creating and maintaining femininity and fertility. Suwen chapter 1, with its full exposition of the seven year cycles of the girl and woman as she commences menstruation, reaches the fullness of her fertility and then moves into menopause, is discussed in depth. There follow sections on infertility, the menopause and various menstrual problems.

While explaining theory and belief in depth this book is also supremely practical and will be of great help in the clinic. It forms a pair with its sister volume Pregnancy and Gestation in Chinese Classical Texts which will be published in the winter of 2007. Together the explanations and insights offered will be of immense help to all those considering and treating women with their 'equal but different' nature.

For the first time in one of our books we are using *qi* only in the plural. This reflects the particular request of Elisabeth Rochat who feels that the plural more accurately reflects the concept of *qi* as it was imagined and experienced by the Chinese at the time of the writing of the majority of texts referred to here. We are also using the older character for *zang/cang* (藏) which does not have the flesh radical and would have been used with both meanings the time of most of these texts.

Translations from the original Chinese are all made by Elisabeth unless otherwise stated. We include Chinese characters throughout for clarity and understanding, and recommend the use of Dr. S. L. Wieger's Chinese Characters (Dover Language Books) for further analysis.

Caroline Root 2007

THE ESSENTIAL WOMAN

In these lectures I propose to look at the specific nature of life in a woman. We will do this by considering blood and qi (氣) and their particular balance in a woman's meridians and organ systems. Afterwards we will look at the main causes of pathology, and will study Suwen chapter 1 to understand the process of development in the body of a girl as she becomes a woman, her ability to make another life, and then her declining fertility. We will also examine menstruation and its main disturbances, infertility and the menopause, looking at texts such as the Jingui yaolüe and the Shanghanlun.

BLOOD AND QI *xue qi* 血 氣

When we speak of women we are speaking of one particular aspect of life within the whole cosmic existence. Life in traditional China was understood as a constant exchange and balance between *yin* (陰) and *yang qi* (陽 氣). This constant exchange is expressed in the human body as blood and *qi* or essences and *qi*. Every living being is a mingling of various *qi* which allow a form to appear. An embryo is the gathering of essences in a concentrating *yin* movement of *qi*. Through these essences and through their knotting together effected by the impulse coming from heaven and giving the potential to develop, there is the beginning of a form and the beginning of the exploration through this form of its specific nature. For each being there is a different impulse or potential which is directed through species, race and lineage. So a child is the result of what comes from and through the parents, but is also full of the initiative and movement of the natural order, or what we may call heaven, *tian* (天). We find this idea particularly expressed in daoist texts from the 3rd century BCE. Every living being not only comes from their parents or from everything which comes through their parents, but also from something which exists behind and beyond all the specific expression of life found in the parents and the lineage. At each level and for each new life, the intrinsic nature is not only the mixture of sperm and blood, man and woman, but also a quality given by heaven. This was the basic belief and theory of traditional China.

The specific qualities which are natural for every individual are not the same for a man and a woman. Studying the ten months of gestation (c.f. Pregnancy and Gestation, Monkey Press, 2007) it seems that in the third month something is decided at the level of the balance of blood and *qi* and from then the sex of the child is determined. In the formation of the embryo the balance and specificity expressed through *yin* and *yang qi* and blood and *qi* are fixed as the basic model of development.

There is a vision of blood and *qi* organizing all the energy and vitality which make human life but doing so in the likeness of life on earth. In the Guanzi chapter 39, a text from the 3rd century BCE, there is a text focusing on earth (*di* 地) and water. A comparison is made between what occurs in nature and what exists inside the human body which is the reverse of what we find in medical books:

> 'Water is the blood and *qi* of earth (*di zhi xue qi* 地之血氣), it is like all that circulates and flows (inside the body) to maintain life and sustain forces (*jin mai* 筋脈).'

Not surprisingly we find the expression blood and *qi* is also used with the meaning of health in general. Another text, from the Chunqiu zuozhuan, Duke Xiang, year 21, speaks of someone concerned about his health:

> 'He has become very skinny, but his blood and *qi* are not yet disturbed.'

This is a way of saying that he may look unwell, but if his blood and *qi* are not disturbed he will be alright. Very often in these texts the blood and *qi* are not really concerned with the physical aspects of life, but rather with the temperament and all the characteristics of mind and will. For instance, to have strength in the blood and *qi* is to have strength in the temper, sometimes too violently. There is a real danger that if we have too much blood and *qi* we may be too warrior-like, and this is especially true for men. Variations in blood and *qi* imply variations in temperament or mood. Excitement by emotion or music can move the blood and *qi*, they are what make reactions.

All these aspects are very interesting when we consider the physiology of a woman because it is so linked with her psychology. There is a very famous text from Confucius's Analects in chapter 16, which speaks of the three ages in the life of a man. Confucius is not talking about physical strength or medicine but about morality, and he is trying to explain that according to the stage of life the blood and *qi* are not the same. There is variation of blood and *qi* and this implies tendencies in the temperament which are not the same. We have to be aware of this in order to know what to correct in our patients and what to be careful of in our life. The Confucian sage is someone who applies himself to morality, good behaviour and so on, and he has to be aware of three things:

> 'Confucius said: There are three things which the superior man guards against. In youth, when the physical powers are not yet settled (*xue qi wei ding* 血氣未定), he guards against lust. When he is strong, and the physical powers are full of vigour (*xue qi fang gang* 血氣方剛), he guards against quarrelsomeness. When he is old, and the animal powers are decayed (*xue qi ji shuai* 血氣及衰), he guards against covetousness.' (Lunyu, XVI, 7, translated by J. Legge)

First, when he is young his blood and *qi* (*xue qi* 血氣)

are not yet stabilized but are in a state of excitement. This is the same in the body of a woman, though with different characteristics. It all relies on the strength of the *qi* of the kidneys (*shen qi* 腎氣) pushing life forward and creating an effervescence in the blood and *qi*. So a young man has to take care about his tendency to be lustful. This is a moral perspective of course!

When he is a little older and more mature, blood and *qi* are in their full vigour, so he has to be aware of quarrels and arguments. It is no longer a question of sexual desire and lust but of the strength inside which says no and opposes another. When the man gets old his blood and *qi* are in decline, and in this case he has to be careful about the desire to obtain or collect things. This is a kind of greed which is explained by understanding that if the life which is blood and *qi* is diminishing, in his inner self there will be a sense of deficiency or fear. Therefore a tendency to acquire and keep things and not let anything get away can develop. A decline in the blood and *qi* is a decline in all the inner vitality made by the surging of the *zang* (藏) and *fu* (府). What we have in the blood and *qi* is a lot more than just a red liquid and an internal movement.

In classical China, in the 1st and 2nd centuries BCE, blood and *qi* were definitely linked with the ability to know or perceive with full consciousness. For instance Xunzi, a Confucian philosopher living in the middle of the 3rd century BCE, cites the example of animals. Animals, and large ones in particular, share having blood and *qi* with humans. This is not the case with vegetation or mineral life:

> 'Among all the living beings (*sheng* 生) between heaven and earth, those having blood and *qi* possess awareness (*zhi* 知).' (Xunzi chapter 19)

The ability to have some kind of inner self, sensitivity, perception, emotion, and consciousness, are all linked with the fact of having blood and *qi*. Xunzi talks about big birds which have more blood and *qi* than small birds and says that when you kill an ant you have no feeling that another ant is grieving for it. But with a larger animal, if it loses its mate, it may come back to haunt the place where they used to be together. Even after a whole season it can come back and make sounds which we take as grief. Even small birds do that, though for a shorter time. The purpose of Xunzi's writing is not medical at all. It is to show that filial piety is something natural for human beings and does not stop with death. We have to continue being filial and respectful with our parents even after they are dead, which is one of the great foundations of Confucianism.

In a lot of texts, for example The Book of Rites, it is said that a human being is composed of blood and *qi* with a heart capable of knowledge or consciousness.

> 'By nature (*xing* 性) a human being possesses blood and *qi*, and a heart that allows awareness (*xin zhi* 心 知). Grief or joy, elation or anger do not stay constantly within [him or her]. They are

reactions to the incitements of [exterior] objects. It is then that the art of the heart (*xin zhu* 心術) intervenes.' (Book of Rites, Yueji)

The various feelings of sadness, joy, elation or anger do not exist continuously inside a person, they appear as a result of influences coming from the exterior. We have to behave according to the Art of the Heart. In a human being everything which is physiology and psychology, tendency and reaction, may be called blood and *qi*.

A human being is ruled by their blood and *qi* and all the variations in the balance between them. But on the other hand a human being is also capable of guiding and ruling the blood and *qi*, and this is called the Art of the Heart. It is very important to know this, because even when we study a woman's physiology or pathology, with all the possible disturbances in feelings and emotions, we must never forget that a women is a human being, so is also able to behave according to the Art of the Heart, and according to the wisdom or discernment which is in her own heart. We are not completely determined by a loss or blockage of blood. Even if there are all these influences on our temperament, there is another level of possibilities which is always present.

We know that what are called blood and *qi* are a lot more than just the substance of the blood and the dynamism of its circulation. They encorporate the whole physiology and all the *yin yang* expression of physiology and psychology, but they also enable the presence of the spirits. The presence of blood means the presence of the spirits and the expression of consciousness, perception and knowledge. It is through our blood and *qi* that we are responsible for our own lives, and if, as is said in Huainanzi chapter 7, we are able to behave in such a way that our five *zang* concentrate and rule our blood and *qi* well, then we will behave correctly, our health will be good and the radiance of life will emanate from us without disturbances.

The balance of blood and *qi* changes according to the age of the person. It also has many other variables and cycles. Any kind of alteration in the external surroundings or internal state will influence the balance of blood and *qi*. For instance the pulses are different according to the seasons and according to variations in the weather. This is stated in Suwen chapter 26 for instance:

'In all acupuncture techniques, one must first observe the *qi* of the sun and moon, of the planets and constellations, of the four seasons (*si shi* 四時) and the eight regulators of time (*ba zheng* 八正); once these *qi* have been decided, one punctures.

Thus, when the weather is warm and the sun shines, man's blood is a rich humour and the defensive *qi* (*wei qi* 衞氣) are floating (superficial, *fu* 浮); then the blood disperses easily and the *qi* circulate easily. If the weather is cold and overcast, man's blood condenses and coagulates and the defensive *qi* are in the depths (*chen* 沉).

When the moon begins to wax, blood and *qi* begin their vitality (essences, *jing* 精) and the defensive *qi* begin to circulate.
When the moon is full, blood and *qi* are in fullness (*shi* 實), the bulk of the flesh is solid.

When it is new moon, the bulk of the flesh weakens, the meridians and connecting network (*jing luo* 經絡) become empty (*xu* 虛), the defensive *qi* leave, the bodily form (*xing* 形) alone remains.
It is therefore according to natural movements (*tian shi* 天時) that one regulates (*tiao* 調) blood and *qi*.'

In cold and warm weather the blood and *qi* do not have the same movement. This is also true of the various phases of the moon, and this is why traditionally some acupuncture schools forbade needling at the new moon, or sometimes at the full moon. During a new moon the blood and *qi* are deep inside and at a low tide. At full moon there is almost an excess because it is a time of maximum expansion, like high tide. So needling could be dangerous for people who are unstable. Of course during the daily cycle of day and night blood and *qi* will also vary, and any activity, physical or mental, will change the balance of blood and *qi*. Life is a continuous change in the balance of *yin yang* as reflected through blood and *qi*.

The particular balance of blood and *qi* in a woman is stated very simply. It is said that for a man *qi* are prevalent and for a woman blood is prevalent. *Qi* are *yang* and blood is *yin*. In the body of a woman there is a natural predominance of *yin* and the *yin* movement of *qi*. This is not a question of quantity. It is not that a woman has more blood than a man. It is more to do with the internal organization of the vital movement of life in the body of a woman where the blood is prevalent and therefore the *yin* movement of *qi* is more prevalent. There is more gathering, descending and concentration taking place in the body of a woman, while there is more expansion and upward, springing movement in the body of a man. It is simply a question of the movement of blood and *qi*, and this is manifest in all the physiology and psychology. For example, the concentrating *yin* movement of the blood will lead to its concentration in the lower abdomen and uterus.

Chong mai and ren mai 衝脈任脈

In the text of Lingshu chapter 65 there is a question about why women do not have beards. The answer given is about the movement of *qi* which leads the blood, because the *qi* is the master and guide of the blood. In the body of a woman the blood is lead by the *yin* movement of concentration, while in a man the blood is lead by the *yang* movement of rising up and springing forth with a diffusing energy.

'*Chong mai* (衝脈) and *ren mai* (任脈) both arise in the middle of the intimate envelopes (or protections, *bao zhong* 胞中). They rise running up the back on the inside and make the sea of the meridians and connective circulations (*jing luo* 經絡). Their pathway, emerged and external, runs along the abdomen on the right and rises. They meet together at the pharynx; a separate circulation (*bie* 別) connects (*luo* 絡) with the lips and the mouth.

When blood and *qi* (*xue qi* 血氣) rise in power, the skin is benefited and the flesh warmed. When only the blood rises in power, a drop by drop infiltration of the layers of the skin gives what is necessary for the growth of the hair.

Now women, in their physiology, have an excess of *qi* and an insufficiency of blood, following the frequent loss of blood; *chong mai* and *ren mai* do not make her mouth and lips flourish (*rong* 榮), and because of this she does not have a beard growing there.' (Lingshu chapter 65)

All these functions are related to the kidneys and the origin, with the kidneys as the mediator of the original power. *Chong* and *ren mai* both start in the middle of the vital envelope or protection (*bao zhong* 胞中), and they rise up the inside of the back and arrive at the sea of the meridians and the network of connections. To be the sea of the *jing* (經) and *luo* (絡) is to be the reservoir for the regulation of all the pathways which allow the circulation of blood and *qi*. Blood and *qi* are ruled and circulated by the meridians and also expressed throughout the body by the connective *luo* (絡) network, which is visible to us as capillaries. But we must not restrict the meaning of a meridian to our understanding of a vein or artery.

When Lingshu chapter 65 says that *chong* and *ren mai* are the sea of the *jing luo* it makes them responsible for everything which organizes the movement of blood and *qi*. After this the text comes to another pathway and another function of *chong* and *ren mai*, which is to be responsible for ruling the surplus of blood and *qi*. This is done by a pathway which is said to rise up on the right side of the abdomen. The right side here serves to indicate that it is guiding the blood, with the blood being *yin* and the right side also being *yin*. The normal pathways of the *chong mai* and the *ren mai* ascend and reach the face. They gather at the level of the throat, and there is a connecting pathway which is said to make a network around the area of the lips and mouth.

The text continues:

> 'When blood and *qi* rise in power, the skin is benefited and the flesh warmed. 'When only the blood rises in power, a drop by drop infiltration of the layers of the skin gives what is necessary for the growth of the hair.'

The skin is full of everything which is able to nourish it, and the flesh is warmed by the presence of the blood and *qi*. Therefore there are not only blood and *qi* but also a surplus of blood, which in the body of a man is directed by the *chong* and *ren mai*. These two meridians run around the lips and the mouth but do not reach the top of the head. This is the reason why in the body of a man they bring all the blood into the lower area of the face. Perhaps the organization of the meridian is here to express life as we observe it from outside? If I scrutinize the body and see that there is a beard or moustache there must be a reason for it, and the reason is that a good use of the superabundance of blood has been made. In this case there is a function expressed by a pathway. For the hair it is another kind of superabundance of blood which we will see later when examining Suwen chapter 1. However the superabundance manifest in the hair is also related to the richness of the kidneys and the dynamism of the liver.

The text continues by saying that women are ruled by a *yin* movement of *qi*, and this is expressed by their prevalence of blood. However, despite this very basic difference from a man in the movement of the *qi* and the prevalence of the *yin*, because of menstruation a woman has a regular loss of blood and so repeatedly experiences another imbalance between blood and *qi*, *yin* and *yang*. This can lead to a lot of pathology.

'Now women, in their physiology (*sheng* 生), have an excess of *qi* and an insufficiency of blood, following the frequent loss of blood; *chong mai* and *ren mai* do not make her mouth and lips flourish (*rong* 榮), and because of this she does not have a beard growing there.'

Chong mai and *ren mai* are responsible for directing the blood downwards and inwards, and not for spreading it upwards and outwards. This means that there is regular blood loss, and lips which do not flourish. We understand, therefore, why *ren* and *chong mai* are so important in the pathology of women because being the ruler and establishing the norm in the balance and distribution of blood and *qi*, they are everything in the physiology of the woman which keeps the balance of blood and *qi* and their movements under control. It is also the blood which makes the richness of the *chong* and *ren mai* and their ability to function.

There is a similar process in psychology where because of the *yin* movement of a woman's *qi* she was seen traditionally as someone naturally in the interior, while a man was by nature more external. In Chinese one name which a man could give to his wife was *nei ren* (內 人, the person who is inside), although I think this is no longer used in mainland China! Of course it is contentious to say that by nature a woman likes to be inside and stay at home. This is the same in every culture including our own, but there is a difficult frontier or borderline between an accurate observation of the movement of life, physiology and cosmology, and social protocols and pressures. There is also a value judgement in the supposition that women are submissive and obedient by nature, so that a woman is only understood to be a real woman if she displays a *yin* temperament. She will also be subject to an excess of *qi* because of her loss of blood, for instance demonstrating anger or repressed anger, jealousy, obsessional thoughts and worries, which in China were emotional qualities very often linked with women. It is not by chance that the character for anger (*nu* 怒) contains the character for woman (*nu* 女).

All this movement of *yin* and *yang* may be observed not only in the physiology, psychology and inner temperament, but also in sexuality and fertility, where for a man the natural movement is a springing up and outwards with an emission and for a woman is a gathering in and a concentration in the inner depths. The problem is that we are not supposed to jump to conclusions or to mix up what is male and masculine or what is female and feminine.

Yin and yang qiao mai 陰陽蹻脈

Sexual differentiation is connected not only with *chong* and *ren mai*, but also with the *qiao mai* (蹻脈). The *qiao mai* are *yin* and *yang*. They are the first *yin yang* couple in the extraordinary meridians, and they show how the balance of blood and *qi* is not the same in the body of a man and a woman, and how the *yang* rules a man and the *yin* a woman. This is stated in

Lingshu chapter 17 which is a chapter dealing with the length of the meridians and their pathways.

Traditionally there was a measurement given for the total length of the meridians in the body, though it did not say if it was the body of a man or a woman. It was a symbolic length because you could not have a measurement which is right for everyone. In the calculation each of the twelve meridians is taken plus *du* and *ren mai* and *yin* and *yang qiao mai*. I do not know why. The problem is that the *yin* and *yang qiao mai* are only counted once, even though they are both bilateral. An explanation is given at the end of Lingshu chapter 17 which says that in fact for a man you add the *yang qiao mai* and for a woman you add the *yin qiao mai*. What is stated is that in the body of a man the *yang qiao mai* is the deep meridian, but the character translated by 'meridian' (*jing* 經) also has the meaning of 'the norm', or the 'rule'.

In the body of a man the *yin qiao mai* plays the role of a *luo* (絡), a connecting meridian, something which depends on another meridian. It is the opposite in the body of a woman, where the *yin qiao mai* creates the norm or the organization, while the *yang qiao mai* is considered as a *luo*, a connection dependant on the *yin qiao mai*. When we consider the *qiao mai* in the body of a woman it is the *yin* which establishes its domination and rule, whereas for a man it is the *yang*. The *qiao mai* are really responsible for the balance of the blood and *qi* in the spaces within the flesh and muscles of the body, just as they are also responsible for the *yin yang* harmony in the succession of day and night and therefore time.

In terms of common pathologies of the *qiao mai* there are two main kinds. One is expressed in Nanjing difficult issue 29, and is to do with problems of contraction, convulsions and so on, which are the result of a bad balance between blood and *qi* in the space of the muscles. Differentiation is made according to the location or according to time, for example if a problem on the leg is on the inner or outer aspect or if on the right or left side, and if the convulsions occur during the day or night.

The second major pathology leading specifically to the *qiao mai* is insomnia and somnolence. These also show a *yin yang* disorder in which they are unable to alternate properly. We rely on the *qiao mai* to regulate the intermingling, blending and harmony of *yin yang*, blood and *qi*. In treatment the two master points of the *qiao mai*, Bladder 62 and Kidney 6, are used, and there are specific rules for dealing with the left and right sides. Certain schools also take different points for men and women.

With the *qiao mai* therefore, there is an understanding of sexual differences which are reliant on different balances of blood and *qi*. For ruling the blood and *qi* there are *chong* and *ren mai*.

BAO LUO 胞絡

Xin bao luo (心包絡) is the system of connections and protections natural and appropriate for the heart. *Bao* (包) and *xin* (心) go together, with *bao* being the protection and *xin* the heart. It is not enough just to be connected, you have to be protected as well. To protect the heart is the same as protecting the surging forth of life, since life reflects the origin and is a question of destiny. The heart has to be able to follow the natural order of life, so we can understand that there is a need for special protection for this place which is the 'heart' of life.

Specific to the body of a woman there is the physical form of the enveloping uterus, with flesh, membranes and blood which protect and connect the new life made inside of her. It is the reason why the character for uterus (*bao* 胞) is the same as the one for the protection of the heart (*bao* 包) but with the radical of the flesh (月) added on the left. So the uterus too has a network of connections. *Bao luo* (胞絡) and *bao mai* (胞脈) are both commonly used expressions for this. *Luo* is connection and *mai* is vital circulation, often concerned with blood. Therefore there are not only the protection and enveloping but also the connection and communication: the entire circulation which allows what is inside the uterus to be nourished and to maintain its form. Even if there is no embryo the state of the uterus itself and the correct maintenance and rhythm of the blood will depend on all the connections maintained between the uterus and other parts of the body, particularly the kidneys. From the heart the network also includes connections from the innermost part of the person to the other *zang fu* and parts of the organism, enabling the distribution of the radiance of the spirits via the blood.

Bao zhong 胞中

Therefore we can understand how the expression *bao zhong* (胞中), the centre of the vital protection, may be used when the *bao* is not related to the heart, and is not translatable as the uterus, and can exist in the body of a man or a woman. It is the place inside each person where life is both protected and connected. The original blueprint and impulse of life are kept safe there to maintain vitality, and the connections and circulations express the power of life. *Bao zhong* is where, as we saw in Lingshu chapter 65, *chong* and *ren mai* start. In later texts it is also given as the starting point of the *du mai* (督脈). We have here the triple expression of life through these three extraordinary meridians, expressing the *yang* with the *du mai*, the *yin* with the *ren mai*, and the powerful merging of the *yin yang* giving blood and *qi* with the *chong mai*. All this expresses the original potential of a life and comes from the place where the quality of *yin yang* and blood and *qi* is decided from the origin.

With the uterus it is very obvious that there is a concentration of blood and its renewal which is able to nourish life, while in the heart there is the starting point of the blood and *qi* giving or offering life to the whole person. It is not by chance that the heart master meridian (also called the *jue yin* of hand or *shou jue yin* 手厥陰) is related to the protection and connections of the heart (*xin bao luo* 心包絡). In Lingshu chapter 10 the heart master meridian is described as responsible for the pathology of the *mai*, the vital circulation and specifically for the movement and circulation of the blood. On the other hand, in Nanjing difficult issues 36 and 39 the protective envelope which is the uterus (*bao* 胞) is linked with the origin and the kidneys, and with the kidneys as *ming men*. *Ming men* (命門) is a place of connection and concentration and relationships with the *yuan qi*, the original *qi*, as said in Nanjing 36. In the body of a man this function is able to keep the essences and form the richness of the sperm. In the body of a woman it is all the connections with the uterus, enabling to blood to enter and nourish it regularly:

> '*Ming men* (命門), it is the residence of the spirits/essences (*shen jing* 神精); it is where the original *qi* (*yuan qi* 原氣) are attached. The man stores (*cang* 藏) the essences (*jing* 精, sperm); the woman attaches the uterus (*bao* 胞).' Nanjing 36

> '*Ming men*, it is the residence of the essences/spirits (vital spirit, *jing shen* 精神). In the man, it stores (*cang* 藏) the essences (*jing* 精, sperm); in the woman, it attaches the uterus (*bao* 胞).' Nanjing 39

There is also a sentence in Suwen chapter 33 which says:

'The circulations of the uterus (*bao mai* 胞脈) depend (*shu* 屬) on the heart and connect (*luo* 絡) with the centre of the vital protection (*bao zhong* 胞中).'

In this context *bao* is the uterus and *mai* are the vital circulations, which means all the network of connections belonging to the uterus. To depend (*shu* 屬) describes the relationship which each meridian has with its own organ. For instance the lung meridian has a *shu* relationship with the lung organ. *Shu* (屬) means to belong to, to be attached to and dependant on, in the way that in feudal times a vassal was linked to his sovereign. *Xin* (心) is the heart, and *luo* (絡) means connections, to connect or to maintain a network of relationship.

The quotation from Suwen chapter 33 therefore tells us that the circulations related to the uterus belong and are attached to the heart, and are also connected with the centre of the vital envelope. This is very interesting because it states a clear difference between *bao* as the uterus and *bao zhong*, the centre of the vital protection. Furthermore, with all the connections, vital circulations and communications extending out from the uterus there is a very deep relationship with the heart and heart protector. This is natural because blood and *qi* really emanate from the heart.

Bao luo 胞絡 and the kidneys

There is also the connection with the original power which is said to be made through the kidneys. Suwen chapter 47 states:

'The connections belonging to the uterus (*bao luo* 胞絡) are attached (*xi* 系) to the kidneys.'

Here the connections are made with and by the kidneys which link up with the origin. This is the same idea as expressed in Nanjing difficult issues 36 and 39, that what is a uterus in a woman has a link with the heart for the blood and with the kidneys for the connection with the original power of life. This association with the kidneys is also a relationship with the function of the kidneys as one of the five *zang*. It is through the kidneys that the connection with the essential nature and power of life is given to the blood in the uterus, and which along with the heart gives the power to nourish another life.

The context of Suwen chapter 33 is the subject of amenorrhoea, and of Suwen chapter 47 is a woman in the ninth month of pregnancy who falls silent and does not speak. It is said that if the woman stops speaking it is because the connecting circulation natural to the uterus (*bao luo* 胞絡) has been interrupted. This is because it is linked to the kidneys and the kidney meridian connects with the root of the tongue. The explanation given is that in the ninth month the weight of the baby becomes too heavy for the woman and it blocks the proper circulation of the kidneys, so therefore they cannot really communicate with the root of the tongue. The woman is exhausted and her kidneys are also exhausted because of this situation. The lack of strength in the kidneys makes the will to speak very weak, and therefore no desire to speak reaches the tongue. Elsewhere in the Suwen the link between the desire to speak and the kidneys is repeated. When a pregnant woman is exhausted and her kidneys are weak with the baby draining all her energy, it is better that she gives all her strength to herself and the baby and not expend it in speech.

Uterus as extraordinary fu

In Suwen chapter 11 the uterus is given as one of the six extraordinary *fu, qi heng zhi fu* (奇恆之府):

'Brain, marrow, bones, vital circulations, gallbladder, uterus, these six are produced by the *qi* of the earth. They store (*cang* 藏) the *yin* and they reflect the image (*xiang* 象) of the earth (*di* 地). Their name is the extraordinary and permanent *fu* (*qi heng shi fu* 奇恆之府).'

We can understand that the uterus is really an extraordinary *fu* because their definition is something which is like a *fu* but functions as a *zang*. (c.f. The

Extraordinary Fu, Monkey Press, 2003) That is to say it is something with an actual space inside, for instance the stomach. This is why they are sometimes called the 'hollow organs' because they have a physical and visible cavity. This is not the case with the *zang* which are a compact mass with no empty space or pocket. The uterus presents as a *fu* (府), but functions as a *zang* (藏), preciously keeping the essences of life inside. This then allows the releasing of *qi* and the functioning of life. The extraordinary *fu* have the ability to deal with the essences and with what is assimilated as useful and vital for the organism, they do not deal with the separation of the essences from waste matter as the proper *fu* do. The gallbladder is an exception to this of course.

The uterus is full of blood, and the blood in the uterus is naturally full of essences and full of the ability to create and sustain a life. This is exactly why the uterus has to keep the blood. You may think that the uterus does not keep the blood because of the regular menstrual loss, but it keeps the blood as long as it is full of life, and eliminates it when it is no longer able to nourish life. The lung does exactly the same thing in the chest when we breathe. In the uterus when the blood is no longer rich enough in essences to make or maintain a new life, the blood has to come out in order to be replaced by fresh blood. In this process the uterus is really acting as an extraordinary *fu*. It alternates between fullness and emptiness in a physical space, but also deals only with the purest and most vital of the substances via the blood of the woman.

Another point worth noting is that in Suwen chapter 11 the uterus of a woman is described as being in a couple with the gallbladder. The gallbladder has several aspects. It is both an ordinary *fu* linked with the liver, but also an extraordinary *fu* full of bile and bile is made of essences which are already assimilated. The gallbladder is not directly part of the digestive tract but it deals with a form taken by the essences. On the other hand the gallbladder also suggests or symbolizes a man's genitals because in the movement of the gallbladder in keeping essences and emitting them there is a reflection of the image of a man's sexuality, keeping and emitting sperm. In Chinese the character for essences, *jing* (精), is very normally used for sperm.

In the double aspect of life in the uterus there is the meeting of the best of the woman's blood, full of the capacity to make and nourish life, and the essences or sperm coming from the man which also have the capacity to generate life. All that is then subject to the natural movement of a woman which is *yin*, to keep, to blend together and to start a form.

ZANG AND FU 藏 府

The *zang* and *fu* are all the organs which together produce the essences and enable the *qi* to make transformations and sustain the production of the blood, thus stimulating the entire operation of life. Good circulation by the *mai* allows the blood to go to the uterus in order to moisten and nourish it and in that way to make conception and nourishment of an embryo possible. Afterwards it ensures a good delivery and the successful production of milk for feeding the baby. Through the functioning of the *zang* a healthy balance of blood and *qi* is maintained, and this is the basis for the correct operation of the body. The *fu* are more dependent on the *zang*, and disturbance at the level of the *fu* can be seen through disturbance in the *zang* or the meridian. The three *zang* which are most important in gynaecology are the kidneys, the liver and the spleen.

The kidneys

In looking at the *zang* we have to start with the kidneys because the kidneys are the basis and foundation of life and therefore the basis and foundation for production of essences. They also give strength to the *qi* and the *yang*, and they allow the *qi* to transform. The kidneys, being the source of the fire and warmth and *qi*, sustain the activity of transformation in all the other organs, and they also have an important role in the production of the blood. The making of blood is based on the liquids which are the expression of the essences, so the kidneys are responsible for the quality of the liquids and essences. In addition the kidneys support all the functioning of the *yang* of the spleen and stomach, and all the proper process of digestion which allows the formation of body fluids. By means of transformation some of these become blood, because blood stems from the liquids coming from the spleen and is completed through the heart. But all of this has to be supported by a strong foundation in the kidneys.

The kidneys are responsible for the individual's relationship with the origin and for the authentic *yin* and *yang* (*zhen yin* 真陰 and *zhen yang* 真陽). This means they ensure the quality of the essences and all the operations of *qi* in all the organs of the body. All posterior heaven is made based on the model of the original life which constitutes anterior heaven. From this perspective the kidneys are responsible for the development and growth of each specific life and for the reproduction of that life. As long as the kidneys are able to maintain the good and full functioning of all the organs, the blood and *qi* will be superabundant and it will be possible to have blood in the uterus with normal menstruation and fertility. It will also be possible to have enough strength and circulation not to have problems during pregnancy or birth, and subsequently to have healthy lactation.

The kidneys are also the source for the relationship

with the origin and the original power of life, and for the resulting fertility. They are the basis upon which the expression of the *chong* and *ren mai* is founded. *Chong mai* and *ren mai* can function fully if the kidneys are able to maintain a sufficient production and movement of blood and *qi*. When this is ensured the *chong* and *ren mai* are able to rule the blood and *qi* in so far as c*hong* and *ren mai* are the specific rulers of the distribution of blood and *qi*. But *chong* and *ren mai* cannot function in this way if the kidneys are not sustaining the renewal of the blood and *qi*. If we do not have properly functioning kidneys and a renewal of vitality, we cannot have fertility.

The kidneys also help balance the *qi* of the heart, as they do in offering pure essences to the heart and allowing the spirits to be present and rule in a person's life according to the natural order. The kidneys maintain and nourish the liver by ensuring that the liver, which is full of blood, stays rooted in the *yin* and the water. The kidneys' relationship with the liver allows this rooting and storing in the depths. The kidneys warm up the spleen, acting in such a way that the spleen benefits from the general fire of life, and its functioning is sustained. They also produce the marrow and nourish the brain. Therefore, because the physiology of a woman is closely linked to the kidneys, if there is tiredness or damage to the kidneys due to pregnancy, delivery or multiple births, there will be symptoms and signs in other organs and on different levels. As we will see in Suwen chapter 1, it is the power coming from the kidneys which allows fertility to begin, which allows menstruation and the *chong* and *ren mai* to function, and which allows the mother's milk to be produced through the stomach and all the other *zang* and *fu*. It also allows very rich blood to come into the uterus and be kept by this activity of storing in the depths, in order to welcome the embryo.

The kidneys are responsible for the inner rhythm of life which is the movement of opening and closing. This is the original rhythm of life, and is perceptible at the level of the abdomen and lower orifices. Something analogous is found in the *wei qi* (衛 氣), the defensive *qi*, which is also responsible for good rhythms and specifically for the good rhythm of opening and closing at the level of the superficial pores. An expression of the kidneys' mastery of the movement to open and close is found in the storing and the letting out from the two lower orifices and the uterus. There is a normal flow in the uterus, with a normal keeping and a normal sending out. But all this depends on the ability of the kidneys to store, to open and to let go. The liver also plays a role of course, but in another way. In this context it is the kidneys and the water element with the ability to attract and keep in the depths, which is the fundamental movement of the *qi* of the water and kidneys. If there is a good balance between the kidneys and the heart, and if there is harmony between *yin* and *yang* in the lower abdomen then there is no weakness or overheating and there is normal sexual desire. The pathology of an excess or a diminution of sexual desire is very linked with the kidneys, although with other organs too of course.

If the kidneys are unable to close and keep something inside there may be leaks, perhaps of urine but also perhaps showing in bleeding or haemorrhage from the uterus. Sometimes there can be an overheating in reaction to this leak and loss of *yin*, and then there may be uncontrollable sexual desire. Lack of *yin* often leads to a reactive heat but also to a weakness in the *yang*, and this in turn results in a deficiency in the quality of the *yin*. If there is a storing or an enclosing which is really a blockage, and there is difficulty in maintaining the rhythm of opening and closing, then there may be a block in urination, or an irregularity in menstruation, with difficulty in the flow of blood. There may also be a diminution of the *yin*, with drying up of the *yin* of the blood, of the genitals, and of the liquids.

Because of the connection of the *du mai* (督脈) with the kidneys, and through the *du mai* the relationship with the brain, when the essences of the kidneys are flourishing and rich and the *qi* of the kidneys is powerful, thought processes will be well sustained along with all the other mental activities which are dependent on the good state of the kidneys. The balance between water and fire, kidneys and heart, is also essential to stabilize the mind, sustain the vital spirits (*jing shen* 精神) and help maintain calm and tranquillity. Avoiding agitation or uncontrollable mental processes relies directly on the communication between kidneys and heart, although the liver is also involved. For instance, if there is an emptiness of the *yin* of the kidneys, there may be liver fire destabilizing the heart. Some kinds of mental disturbance, either agitation or despondency or loss of memory, are also often linked to tiredness of the kidneys. Psychosomatic problems and the disturbance of menstruation are similarly connected. We understand this from a western approach, but from the Chinese perspective it is not simply a question of psychosomatic symptoms but of a disturbance of menstruation and mind explained by the poor functioning of the organs.

The liver

The liver stores the blood. But the double aspect of the liver means that at the same time it masters the releasing of blood, the flowing out and putting in motion which is the impulse given to all movement and circulation. We can say that these are two different functions of the liver, but this is not exactly true. It is the movement of the liver on the *yin* side storing the blood, and on the *yang* side giving the impulse for all circulation, sending forth and spreading out. As always the *yin* is the basis for the *yang*. It is only because the liver is able to keep the blood that it is also able to give the correct strength to all the outward moving impulses and circulations.

This is particularly important in a woman's physiology. First there is the *yin* activity of keeping the blood, with the gathering and storing of the blood in the uterus. Second, there is the liver's function of sending forth, *shu xie* (疏 泄). *Shu* (疏) means to be relaxed and at ease without any tension, but at the same time the character means to spread out and clear out, so there is the idea of clearing the way. The general meaning of *shu* is that there is no obstacle to movement in the circulation, no tension, tightening or pressure. At the same time the movement is well-balanced. Everything flows easily with enough strength, even at the origin, to go right up to the edge. This relates to the specific movement of the liver as a spring, giving an impulse.

Xie (泄) means to flow out. It is used for water flowing and leaking out. *Xie* may also be used for perspiration or diarrhoea. This is not the meaning here. This is more an oozing or leaking out, with the idea of flowing out in a spreading way. The strength of the *yang* is based on the storing of the blood, but it must be a very balanced and nourished strength which allows the liver to give a controlled impulse to circulate and spread everywhere. This is exactly the double movement which we have at all levels of physiology and psychology. The blood which is kept by the liver is kept in order to be set free. There is no point of keeping something for the sake of keeping it. It is kept to have an effect.

The liver is involved in the distribution of the blood in a different way from the heart. The heart is responsible for the very regular circulation of the blood, the movement which is linked with the vital circulations, the *mai*, and which spreads along the pathways unceasingly.

Associated with the liver is the natural movement of the wood, which is a concentration to the point of opening up and letting go. This is a dynamic movement which is different from the opening and closing which are an effect of the keeping in the depths. With the liver the storing is done in order to be able to release. As far as blood itself is concerned the releasing of blood enables the muscular forces to work by discharging blood in the muscles in order to let them move. This is also true for menstruation because the alternating rhythm of blood being kept and then sent forth is another expression of the liver. We can see therefore why the liver has such an important role in menstruation and in the quantity of blood flowing out. If the liver is overexcited or there is fire in the liver, there will be an inability to keep the blood, causing excessive flow or even haemorrhage.

As usual with the liver many blockages are due to emotions and psychological disturbances in which the emotion and the internal chaos are not able to be cleared out. We cannot 'clear out' our inner disposition if we are not able to relax and have normal circulation in our mind and feelings. This leads to blockage of the liver *qi* by the emotions, and emotional disturbance is always a kind of inability to release. This is different from the type of obsessive thinking which we see with the spleen.

The liver meridian runs through the whole lower abdomen and around the bladder and genitals. This shows that the same movement of the liver which results in the concentration and expelling of blood from the uterus also makes the urine flow out. Quite often there can be joint disturbances and irritation of the urinary tract at the time of menstruation which are symptoms associated with the liver.

The liver meridian is also linked with the spleen and stomach, particularly at the level of the legs, but in the abdomen there is also a connection with the spleen and stomach meridians as well as the close proximity of the organs. The liver meridian goes through the stomach and all these connections explain very generally the pathological relationships between wood and earth, liver, gallbladder and spleen and stomach which play a large role in gynaecology. There is obviously a lot of pathology related to the liver which is explained by its relationship with the stomach. For example, an imbalance of blood and *qi* at the beginning of a pregnancy can cause a counter current in the stomach which is the cause of the nausea in morning sickness.

The liver meridian directly connects to the stomach meridian through the chest and breast. The stomach and the liver are both very involved in lactation. The stomach is more in charge of making the liquids, while the liver is involved with exactly the same movement we have just seen of keeping and releasing. This is also a good help in spreading and clearing out in case of blocked lactation. The pathology of lactation which is linked with the liver arises in the form of blockages not in problems with quantity. All this relates to the harmony of the *qi* and the *yin yang* of the liver at the level of the lower abdomen and with the help given to the spleen and stomach at the level of the chest.

Relationships between liver and heart are important

in the balance and calm of a woman's psychology. Very often anger is associated with a woman's menstruation because the regular loss of blood endangers the balance in her liver. The loss of blood creates a situation where at least during certain days there is not enough blood to compensate for the strength of the liver. Therefore an imbalance occurs and psychologically this can manifest as anger. If the anger is not expressed, because of the prevalence of the *yin* in the woman, then you can have a blockage of the *qi* of the liver with agitation and other characteristics such as jealousy and suspicion. The character for anger is *nu* (怒): a woman (女) is depicted with a heart underneath (心). On the right side is a right hand (又), so the woman is a slave (奴) because the hand is the hand of the master, and anger is the feeling of a woman repressed by her master.

One of the other names given to the liver is the sea of blood (*xue hai* 血海). But this is also a title used for the uterus and the *chong mai*, as stated in Lingshu chapter 33. Some books even say that blood is so important for a woman that the liver is her anterior heaven. For a man the kidneys remain the anterior heaven, linked to the essences which are the sperm. This observation is just to make it clear that it is due to the liver that the blood is able to make life.

Between the functions of the kidneys and the liver is the ancestral muscle, the converging place of all the muscular forces, the *zong jin* (宗筋). The meaning of this expression is something equivalent to ancestral *qi* (*zong qi* 宗氣), the place where all the *qi* converge in the sea of *qi* in the middle of the chest in order to establish their correct rhythm and quality. In the same way the ancestral muscle is the place from which the quality and strength of all muscular movements is ruled. It has a special relationship with the tendino-muscular pathways, since several of them converge with the liver tendino-muscular:

> '[The liver tendino-muscular] ...makes a knot (*jie* 結) at the genitals where it connects (*luo* 絡) with all the tendino-muscular (*jin* 筋).' (Lingshu chapter 13)

The *zong jin* (宗筋) is a place where everything which rules and belongs to the muscular forces gathers and shows correct functioning, for example how the liver is able to send the blood supporting the *qi* to the muscles to make movement. This is a very general interpretation, and at this level there is an ancestral muscle in the bodies of both men and women. But the expression is also used more specifically for the muscles responsible for an erection in a man. However the *zong jin* is important for a woman too, because in the area of her lower abdomen it demonstrates the strong presence of the liver with all its ability to make the muscular forces which are so important in delivery. Usually the name *zong jin* is not used in this context but rather with specific reference to a man. Nevertheless, the role of the liver and the muscular forces is very important for the muscles of the lower abdomen in both men and women, and in this area there will always be an important link between the liver and the kidneys.

The meeting and gathering together of the liver meridian and *ren mai* occurs at the level of the lower abdomen and uterus, specifically at Ren 2 (*qu gu* 曲骨). It is very interesting to see the liver meridian not only uniting with *ren mai* in the lower abdomen, but also with *du mai* at the vertex of the head, the place around which the hair starts growing, Du 20 (*bai hui* 百會). The meridian helps the blood to go upwards to nourish the whole head and hair.

Question: Did the ancient Chinese understand the functioning of the ovaries?

No. I have not seen any ancient text which demonstrates an understanding of what we know nowadays as the ovaries. But they were not so interested in anatomical descriptions. They were interested in describing function. They did have names for the pancreas and other parts of the body, and when they opened up animals they saw the organs, so it is not a question of not knowing about them, but they were not interested in them. Part of the explanation may be that those things did not make sense in the same way that their perception of the movement of life made sense and sustained their understanding of diagnosis and choice of treatment.

Spleen and stomach

As the root of posterior heaven the spleen and stomach are the source from which blood and *qi* are created through transformation. The spleen is in charge of transporting and transforming the liquids and grains and transporting all the essential nutriments coming from digestion and assimilation. In doing this it nourishes the whole body and sustains the renewal of all the body fluids (*jin ye* 津液). From these comes the substance which forms the basis of the blood and milk. Another function of the spleen is to transform damp, and it is responsible for the management of the damp and liquids which are so important in the *yin* body of a woman. Bad transformation of damp can result in vaginal discharges for example.

The nourishment of the blood and the transportation of the nutriments essential for the maintenance of the embryo and the creation of milk all depend on the capacity of the spleen to reproduce blood and *qi* successfully. The spleen must be able to renew the substance of the blood making it not too thick and not too thin. The spleen also sustains the activities of the other organs by nourishing them so that these organs release their *qi*. The good strength of the *qi* in the organism is dependent on the good functioning of the spleen, which is the source of blood and *qi* and the foundation of posterior heaven. If the balance of blood and *qi* is good then the blood can follow its own course. If the blood remains inside its own pathways of circulation this reflects the important function of the spleen of keeping the blood in the right place, which is due to the strength of the *qi* of posterior heaven. All of this is very important in gynaecology, both in menstruation and during pregnancy, and also during delivery. In addition it is about keeping the uterus in the right place because the spleen *qi* ensures the correct rising up movement.

If we consider the stomach more specifically, the *yang ming* meridian is rich in blood and *qi*. There are strong relationships between the stomach meridian and *chong mai* as discussed in Nanjing difficult issue 27 for instance, where their pathways are taken together. There are also strong relationships between the *chong mai* and the kidney meridian, with the points of the kidney meridian in the lower abdomen generally given as points of the *chong mai*. This is found in Suwen chapter 60. This togetherness of the pathways related to the kidneys and the stomach indicates a common function which concerns the *chong mai*, that is the relationship with the origin providing the original nature and pattern of life and its expression and development inside an individual.

In the deep relationship between the stomach and *chong mai* the concern is the richness of the sea of blood. The stomach is sometimes called the sea of blood, or sea of blood and *qi*, and *chong mai* is also a sea of blood. The blood of *chong mai* is reliant on the capacity of the stomach to renew all blood and *qi*. This is stated in Suwen chapter 44. The blood which is under the rule of the *chong mai* comes from the healthy functioning of the stomach and spleen. Zhang jiebin said the blood of the *chong mai* also comes from the transformation of liquids and grains through the *yang ming* and the *qi* of the stomach. So these are the basis for the *chong mai*.

There is in addition a deep relationship between the stomach and *ren mai* (任 脈). For instance, from Ren 10 to Ren 13 the *ren mai* actually passes through the stomach, supporting the *mu* point of the stomach at the level of Ren 12 (*zhong wan* 中 脘). All the *yin* renewed by the stomach or the essences assimilated through the work of the stomach, create the basis for the proper functioning of the *ren mai*. When the stomach works well, blood and *qi* are sufficient, the sea of blood is full and lactation is rich. The *yang ming* stomach meridian is involved in lactation and the formation of the liquids in a mother's milk. We can see, therefore, that there is always a vision of the spleen and stomach as the root of everything which is renewed in the body, and in classical gynaecological treatises it says that menstruation as well as a mother's milk come from the spleen and stomach.

The spleen meridian has a special relationship with the *ren mai* meridian at the level of Ren 3 (*zhong ji* 中 極) in the lower abdomen. The spleen has the ability to maintain things in their correct place, and also to make the clear, the pure and the essences rise upwards. It has the capacity to make sure that what is essential and vital is not lost via haemorrhage or diarrhoea. By the same movement of keeping in the right place and rising up, the spleen has a role in the maintenance of the organs of the abdomen, and a specific role in uterine prolapse. For the spleen and stomach, each time there is something lacking concerning food or nutrition, such as a bad or insufficient diet, or difficulty in assimilation and digestion, the quantity of blood will suffer. In the extreme case of famine, there may be resulting amenorrhoea. They certainly have experience of this in China.

Question: What about vaginal mucus?

This is to do with the body fluids and their pathology. In general body fluids leaking out via the uterus is a sign that there is a lot of damp in the lower abdomen. But body fluids do a lot of smoothing, irrigating and nourishing as well. However, I know of no text which talks about vaginal mucus helping the process of fertilization or indicating the time of fertility.

The heart

There are many relationships between the heart and the blood, or between the heart and the blood's circulation. The following sentences are frequently found in different texts:

'The heart masters the blood (*xin zhu xue* 心主血).'
'The heart masters the vital circulations (*xin zhu mai* 心主脈).'

'The heart masters the blood circulations (*xin zhu xue mai* 心主血脈).'

The heart is *xin* (心), *zhu* (主) is to master, *xue* (血) is blood, *mai* (脈) is vital circulations perceptible at the pulses. Every kind of circulation is *mai*, a meridian is *mai*, a *luo* is *mai*. But *mai* linked to the heart show how these circulations come from the heart's pulsation sending a rhythmic impulse for circulation, and more specifically blood circulation, throughout the body. It is the good quality of the *yin yang* balance in the blood and *qi* which allows this regular movement. If we do not have harmony at the level of the *yin yang* of the heart we do not have any regular beating or pulsation within the body.

All these circulations with the right rhythm and movement are perceptible on the pulse. This is why the character *mai* is also used to mean the pulse. We can understand therefore how and why the heart masters the *mai*, and why it is not quite possible to translate *mai* here as pulse. The heart masters all the circulations which are continuously moving in the body by means of the regular rhythm it gives. When the heart is said to master the blood, the blood is only called blood after having undergone changes and transformations as it finally passes through the heart.

The blood not only has an irrigating and nourishing power, but also the ability to warm. Above all it is the substance through which the spirits, or consciousness, travel inside the body from the heart to the periphery and back again. This is stated in many texts, both in the Neijing and elsewhere. The blood is said to be the dwelling place of the spirits, so when we say the heart masters the blood circulation (*xue mai* 血 脈) it means that the heart masters all the circulations carrying the blood. *Xin zhu* (心 主), the heart masters or the heart as a master, is the name normally given in Chinese to the meridian which we usually call the *jue yin* of the hand.

When the heart correctly masters the blood and all the blood circulations (which is not the same as the circulation of blood described in modern Western medical books) it implies the necessity of a centre and something moving from it. It is unthinkable that the blood does not move. Blood has to move all the time and the movement has to be centred, and ruled from the centre which is the heart. The circulation is how blood spreads everywhere throughout the body but remains under the control of the heart.

When the heart works well all the connections of the *mai* with the uterus participate in helping the blood go to the uterus. As we saw earlier in the quotation from Suwen chapter 33:

> 'When the menses do not come, the reason is that the circulations of the uterus (*bao mai* 胞 脈) are closed (*bi* 閉). The *bao mai* (胞 脈) depend on the heart and are connected with the *bao zhong* (胞 中, centre of the vital protections or envelopes), the original vital centre. When the *qi* rise up and make a pressure against the lung, the *qi* of the

heart can no longer descend easily. This is the reason why the menses do not come.'

In this example it is in the context of an inner heat coming from an emptiness of the kidneys. This explains the counter current of the *qi* blocking the lung and preventing the descending movement of the heart. The kidneys and the heart no longer communicate, so there is a lack of normal blood circulation irrigating the lower abdomen and nourishing the uterus.

The vital circulations going to the uterus are dependent on the heart. Any disturbance in the heart may have an effect on menstruation or on the movement of life inside the woman. The disruption can be physical or psychological.

In Suwen chapter 44 there is an example given of a disturbance due to emotion. Sadness blocks the *qi* of the chest, tightening it and preventing proper circulation of the blood from the heart. Heat is generated by the blockage so that when there is a crisis the inner heat pushes the blood and the blood descends in the form of uterine haemorrhage. For the man it would cause haematuria, blood in the urine.

'In case of intense sadness and affliction (*bei ai* 悲哀), the protective envelopes and connective network [of the heart] (*bao luo* 胞絡) are interrupted (*jue* 厥). Hence the *yang qi* (陽氣) start to move in the interior (*nei* 內). When the illness is set off, the heart causes haemorrhages (metorrhagia) below and there is frequent blood in the urine (haematuria).'

These are just two examples from the Neijing of the importance of the heart as the general master of the whole blood circulation. If the blood does not circulate properly then the liver is affected as well as the kidneys and all other parts of the body. In a woman this will be felt immediately in the lower abdomen, the uterus and in menstruation.

The lung

What is fundamentally important about the lung is that it masters the *qi*, and one of the aspects of this mastering is the rhythm and movement of *qi* which gives the impulse to the vital circulations, *mai*. Suwen chapter 21 talks about the lung receiving the one hundred *mai* at the morning audience. This means that at dawn, at the time when everything is in the best possible state of balance because of the night's rest, the lung is able to start the daily distribution of circulation once again on a fresh basis and in good balance. This is done at the time belonging to the lung meridian in the early morning before the beginning of the day's activities, so that there is the best possible balance in the *qi* gathering in the chest and lung. The morning audience of the lung for the one hundred *mai* offers the best possible rhythm to the chest and heart and the circulations of blood and *qi*. It is one of the ways that good functioning of the lung and the *qi* of the lung is helpful for all the circulation and regulation of the blood.

There is not only a movement of spreading out coming from the lung, but also a pressure to make things such as water descend. The lung makes liquids in the trunk go down to the bladder. In the descending movement of the lung we have help given to the circulation of the blood descending to the uterus. There is a balance between the lung and the kidneys, and there is a balance between the lung and heart at the level of blood and *qi* and the rhythm of the circulation and movement of *qi*. But we also have a relationship between the lung and the kidneys which is visible in respiration, where the kidneys help the descent of the breath.

In gynaecology what is more important is the link between the lung and the kidneys as far as the body liquids are concerned. The balance of liquids and *qi* inside the lung is very important because if we have an imbalance, for example not enough liquids or inner heat, whatever is wrong in the lung may disturb lactation and also the liver and stomach meridians passing through the chest. So the lung is important because of its connections with the heart, kidneys, liver and stomach.

THE EXTRAORDINARY MERIDIANS

Chong mai 衝脈

The *chong mai* (衝脈) begins inside the vital envelope (*bao zhong* 胞中) at the origin of life. Together with the kidneys and the stomach meridians it passes through the lower abdomen and upwards through the stomach, diffusing in the chest and moving up to the throat. The *chong mai* plays an important role in the ways in which blood is distributed throughout the body, in both centrifugal and centripetal movements depending on whether it is in a man or a woman. The *chong mai* is in a relationship with the kidneys making the link with anterior heaven, and is associated with the stomach and the *yang ming* meridian of the stomach to maintain and nourish the essences and *qi* coming from posterior heaven. It is also connected with the kidneys to benefit the kidney *yang*, not only with regard to the essences and the blood of posterior heaven but also to ensure the gentle warmth of the original fire and the proper care and protection of the essences coming from the authentic *yin* and *yang* of the kidneys and *qi* of anterior heaven.

Chong mai therefore has a kind of bridging function, and this enables the balance of blood and *qi* which is natural for each gender. There is also a relationship with the liver because the connection between the liver and the *chong mai* allows the *chong mai* to rule the superabundance of blood, which at an organ level is taken charge of by the liver. The liver stores the blood and releases it, working with the superabundance of blood. The *chong mai* is the extraordinary meridian which regulates the circulation of blood and *qi* through all the meridians and *luo*, as seen in Lingshu chapter 65. But the *chong mai* also rules the 'extra' blood and *qi* and is responsible for guiding it in the right direction. In Chinese they say that the *chong mai* also receives the blood of the liver to regulate the nourishment and maintenance of the body. This is the reason why *chong mai* is called the sea of the five *zang* and six *fu*, and the sea of the twelve meridians and *luo* as well as the sea of blood.

All this is perceptible in the pathology of the *chong mai* which is given in the Nanjing and Neijing. For example, in Suwen chapter 60 and Nanjing difficult issue 29 it says that a counter current in the *qi* and a heaviness or stagnation in the lower part of the trunk are the double aspect of pathology of the *chong mai*. Normally *chong mai* gives the correct direction to the *qi*, and since the *qi* guides the blood the *chong mai* is thus ensuring the proper diffusion of the blood throughout the lower part of the body avoiding stagnation and masses. Therefore it is easy to see the role of the *chong mai* in menstruation. But it is also important for lactation because of the relationship with *yang ming* and the use of the richness of the *yang ming*, and its action of diffusing in the chest.

As we will see in Suwen chapter 1, *chong mai* is also very important for fertility. *Chong mai* has the ability to guide the *qi*, and the blood via the *qi*, and thereby it ensures the link between the essences of anterior heaven and the essences of life inside the blood. The *chong mai* is really a way of being able to make the right movement with the right quality of essences and blood in the body of a woman, and this allows fertility so that a pregnancy can start and continue.

Ren mai 任脈

The *ren mai* (任脈) begins alongside the *chong mai* and *du mai* in the place of connection with the origin through the kidneys. So the *ren mai* runs through the lower abdomen with a very strong relationship with the origin and with the three *yin* meridians of the liver, spleen and kidneys, the three most important *zang* in gynaecology. Of course the relationship with the kidneys is particular strong, especially at Ren 4 (*guan yuan* 關元). We also know that the two seas of *qi* are located on the *ren mai*, one on the lower abdomen and one in the middle of the chest. The *ren mai* also masters all the expression of *yin* in the body, this includes the *yin* meridians but also the essences and all the forms they take through the blood, the liquids and so on. Essences, blood and bodily fluids are all under the authority of the *ren mai* because the *ren mai* checks and sustains their good quality and quantity for use in all the manifestations of *yin* and essences in the body. *Ren mai* is the basis of everything which nourishes and maintains the blood and essences, so the *ren mai* has a very specific role in ensuring the quality of the *yin* able to nourish an embryo during gestation for example.

Wang Bing, a great editor and commentator on the Suwen from the Tang Dynasty said that the *ren mai* masters the uterus and the embryo during gestation. Certainly the translation of *ren mai* (任脈) as 'conception vessel' came from this understanding. But it is not a very accurate translation because the *ren mai* exists in the body of a man with essentially the same function as in a woman. In a woman the *ren mai* acts even when she is not pregnant, although when she is pregnant it certainly acts more. In fact the *ren mai* receives and manages the essences and the blood coming from the common work of the *zang* and shares this responsibility for their nourishment and good management with the *chong mai*. The *chong mai* specifically provides the good balance of the blood and *qi*, of the *yin* and *yang*, and of all the dynamism in the movement and circulation of blood and essences. But *chong* and *ren mai* are linked together for the fertility and preservation of the woman's body.

Du mai 督脈

Du mai is important in gynaecology, just as *ren mai* is important in the body of a man. Even if we only consider the meridian of the *du mai* up the back, taking the simplest pathway from Du 1 to Du 28, we can see that *du mai* is a support for the *yang*. It makes the strength of the circulation of the perineal flow, influencing everything which is able to hold up the organs and sustaining the *yang* in each of them, particularly in the area of the lower abdomen. The same thing happens at the level of the chest, where the *du mai* helps the function of the lung. *Du mai* ensures the presence of the authentic *yang*, which permits the renewal of *qi* and strength in connection with the original *yang*. *Du mai* guarantees the presence of the most authentic *yang* at each level of the trunk, and in particular in the lower abdomen. The strength of the *qi* and all their various activities, the warming of the organs and the proper functioning of the body all depend on the *yang qi*.

Suwen chapter 60 has a presentation of the *du mai* describing a pathway inside the abdomen. This emphasizes the importance of the *yang* within the *yin*. As far as we can tell, the vision of the body in traditional China always had the *yang* within the *yin* and the *yin* within the *yang*. This is the way it worked, and therefore in the midst of the *yin* area of the lower abdomen there is a strong presence of *yang* expressed in the fire of *ming men* in the lower heater, and in the presence of *du mai*. The presence of *du mai* in the lower abdomen is very important in making certain of the warming dynamism and movement to prevent cold, which is one of the main causes of disease and disturbance in gynaecology.

You may ask what is the difference between this and the circulation coming from the liver or the *yang* of the kidneys? There is no real difference. When we label things meridians or extraordinary meridians it is simply a way to gather functions together. The *du mai* is responsible for the organization and settling of the *yang* coming from the origin, and the *ren mai* does the same for the *yin*. When we look at the *zang* we see at how these functions are shared between them, each with its own specific energy and movement of *qi*. The *yang* which is controlled by the *du mai* is not a different *yang* from the one we find associated with the liver or the kidneys, and the warming of the spleen by the *du mai* is the same thing as the gentle warming of the spleen by the kidneys. It is the same thing but seen from another perspective. It is because there is this deep association between *du* and *ren mai*, and the harmony between *yin* and *yang* that anything is possible and that menstruation and fertility work well.

Dai mai 帶脈

Finally we need to speak about the *dai mai* (帶脈). *Dai mai* is based at the level of *ming men*, Du 4. It appears at the extremity of the last rib in the area of the liver points Liver 13 and 14, and moves through the body with the gallbladder meridian, connecting specifically at Gallbladder 26, 27 and 28. It envelopes the body like a girdle, with a containing movement. But it is not just a belt around the body, it is a function which exists everywhere in that area. It contains and holds together all the meridians, which means it rules the rising and descending movements and it circulates to control and normalize the exchanges between up and down. This pivotal role is guaranteed by its connections with the gallbladder meridian.

It is very obvious that when the *dai mai* lacks strength not enough support is given to the rising up movement in particular, and therefore there are descending symptoms, such as descending of liquids resulting in leakages and vaginal discharges. Damp which is not well transformed will also lead to another kind of vaginal discharge. The name for these discharges is *dai xia* (帶 下). *Xia* (下) means to descend and *dai* (帶) is the belt or girdle which gives its name to the extraordinary meridian. In some books *dai* is the traditional name for gynaecology or gynaecological pathology. *Dai xia* is a name which can be given to any kind of gynaecological disease but nowadays it is used specifically for vaginal discharges.

SUWEN CHAPTER 1

Nearly everything which we saw in relation to the five *zang* and the extraordinary meridians helps us to understand this text. Chapter 1 of Suwen consists of two parts with a conclusion on the nature of being human which means to become a sage and an authentic man. First, there is Huangdi's question about why human beings die before they reach one hundred years old. He asks why are they unable to live their lives up until this age without a decline in activity, and whether this is because the natural order, or laws of nature as understood by the ancient Chinese, have changed, or because human beings are behaving badly? The answer given is that it is because of bad behaviour.

Due to the political turmoil of the times, in the 3rd century BCE the Chinese vision of the universe had the idea of an evolution within the natural cycle. The natural order was the movement of life, and there were variations in that natural order according to different cycles. This is how changes in ruling dynasties were explained. The ancient Chinese had the perspective that there were shifts in the natural order but that they were part of a greater order. Relating this to the body they saw there was a constant change in the internal balance, with differences arising according to the time of day or time of year. This is the basis of the cycle of the five elements.

The second part of Suwen chapter 1 concerns the question of the transmission of life and fertility. Huangdi says that at a certain age fertility arrives and a person is able to procreate. But this ability to make life and generate another living being stops before the end of an individual's life, so is this the result of bad behaviour or is it a natural law? The answer to this is that it is a natural law and part of the natural order. The capacity to give life is not the same as the length of a life.

The conclusion of Suwen chapter 1 is not a dialogue between Qi Bo and Huangdi, it is just a declaration by Huangdi and a presentation by the sage about the perfect human being. There are four categories of human beings: those with the power of the universe, those on the way to becoming perfect, sages who are still involved in the world, and lastly, experts who are nearly the same as the sages. These individuals have a real knowledge of things and are able to express this knowledge and help the rulers and doctors and so sustain their activity in the world by means of their accurate knowledge of the natural order. With the first two categories we do not know if they ever exist in the world or not, but sages are not disturbed by the world and its fluctuations.

Seven and eight year cycles

In the second part of the chapter it states that there is a natural law giving a normal beginning and end to the ability to have children. This natural law is then elaborated, first for a woman progressing in periods of seven years, and afterwards for a man with periods of eight years.

Seven is the number of *shao yang* (少陽), the young *yang*, and eight is the number of the *shao yin* (少陰), the young *yin*. This is taking the *shao yin* and *shao yang* as they are used in the Book of Change, not as the meridians of the body which we usually associate with them. In the Book of Change *shao yin* and *shao yang* are part of the four images (*si xiang* 四象), which are young *yang*, young *yin*, old *yang* (*tai yang* 太陽) and old *yin* (*tai yin* 太陰). One of the most obvious examples of these are the four seasons: the *tai yin* is the winter, the *tai yang* the summer, the *shao yang* the spring and *shao yin* the autumn. This perspective is quite different from the use of these expressions as related to meridians.

The body of a woman and her whole physiology is predominantly *yin* and has more to do with the building and achievement of a form, while on the other hand a man has more to do with *qi* and initiating a process. In sexual union there is the start of a process involving the sending and receiving of sperm and then the slow building and achieving of something. This is also the interplay of heaven and earth as represented in a man and woman by sexual intercourse. Seven and eight were used in treatises on sexuality and eroticism.

Seven and eight are numbers which were linked to the balance of *yin* and *yang* in ancient times. There are references to this in several books, and even in the Suwen other chapters, for example chapter 5, allude to seven's power to decrease and eight's to increase:

'If one knows the seven decreasings and eight increasings (*qi sun ba yi* 七損八益) one is able to regulate (*tiao* 調) both (i.e. *yin* and *yang*). But acting without this knowledge leads only to a premature decline.'

In the context of Suwen 1 we can count seven periods of decline: three for a woman (five times seven years, six times seven years, seven times seven years) and four for a man (five times eight years, six times eight years, seven times eight years, eight times eight years). There are also eight periods of prosperity and development: four for a woman (seven years, two times seven years, three times seven years, four times seven years) and four for a man (eight years, two times eight years, three times eight years, four times eight years).

More generally, this expression of increasing and decreasing is used for the balance of *yin yang*, especially related to sexuality and reproduction of life. Seven and eight are another way to look at the movement of *yin* and *yang* and their balance in the body. However, the question as to why there is a *yang* number, seven, linked with women is often asked. Why not have a *yin* number to reflect a woman's *yin* nature? The reason is that you need the dynamism of the *yang* inside the body of a woman in order to make things evolve.

The text of Suwen chapter 1 continues with the Emperor asking a question:

'Men (and women) beyond a certain age have no

children. Is it their power (*cai* 材) that has run dry? Or is it rather the effect of law (*shu* 數) fixed by heaven?'

The answer given is not simply 'It is the natural order of things', but the meaning is essentially the same:

'In a woman of seven years the kidney *qi* (*shen qi* 腎氣) rises in power (*sheng* 盛), the teeth are renewed and the hair grows longer.

At two times seven years fertility (*tian gui* 天癸) arrives, *ren mai* (任脈) functions fully (*tong* 通) while the powerful *chong mai* (衝脈) rises in power (*sheng* 盛). The menses flow downwards in their time (*shi* 時) and she has children (*you zi* 有子).

At three times seven years the kidney *qi* is even (*ping jun* 平均), then the wisdom teeth grow vigorously.

At four times seven years the muscles and bones (*jin gu* 筋骨) are very firm (*jian* 堅), the hair reaches its greatest length, the body becomes powerful and strong.

At five times seven years the circulations (*mai* 脈) of the *yang ming* decline (*shuai* 衰), the face begins to wrinkle, the hair begins to fall.

At six times seven years the three *yang mai* begin their decline above, the whole face wrinkles, the hair begins to whiten.

At seven times seven years the *ren mai* is empty (*xu* 虛) and the powerful *chong mai* declines progressively; fertility dries up. Nothing further passes through (*tong* 通) the way of earth (*di dao* 地道). The body withers and she no longer has children.'

Reference is made here several times to the kidney *qi*. In this context kidney *qi* is not what is called kidney *qi* in usual presentations of TCM, where it refers specifically to the *yang* of the kidneys. In this text kidney *qi* is used to indicate both the *yang* and the *yin* of the kidneys and all their normal functioning. Therefore we have to understand 'kidney *qi*' as designating the expression of the relationship with the origin and its potential throughout the whole body. This potential is realized through the mediation of the kidneys, but only in cooperation with all the other organs.

No other *zang* is mentioned in this passage in Suwen chapter 1. The liver appears at the very end of the whole presentation in relation to the fertility of a man, but there is no detailed functioning of the organ given. We only have the foundation upon which other organ functioning is based. This is the strength and quality coming from the origin, the warmth of the original fire, and the nutrition and irrigation rooted in the model of the original water. This is the meaning of what is called the authentic *yin* and *yang* of the kidneys in later texts. The 'kidney *qi*' therefore represent all of this.

We see the internal working of the kidney *qi* by means of the visible manifestations of the body, and traditionally two of the best places to see it are in the hair and the teeth. This is the reason why hair and teeth are mentioned all the time in this passage in Suwen chapter 1. It is not to focus specifically on the hair and teeth but because they indicate the inner functioning of the kidneys. Teeth show the strength of the *yang* of the kidneys as do the bones, and hair shows the richness of the essences of the kidneys, as does the marrow.

Seven years old

At seven years old 'the teeth are renewed and the hair grows longer.' This means that a little girl of seven years has the possibility of using the vital strength coming from her kidneys for more than just growing up and developing her own body, which was the case up until this age. Previously she matured according to the model sustained by the kidneys, growing normally with the necessary firmness, without delays, weaknesses or malformations. The kidneys work to give richness to the marrow in order to give strength to the bones, and also to give richness to the marrow of the brain. This gives the ability to use the sense organs with precision.

Little by little there was also the building of the vital

spirits (*jing shen* 精神) by means of the connection with the heart. The foundation of the heart was able to benefit the kidney essences and the essences coming from the other *zang*, and all the knowledge and memories built up by the sense organs functioning via a richly nourished brain. The whole strength and force of the kidneys were used to do that, so at around seven years old there is something which is achieved, not complete yet, but achieved in the solidity of the bones, the growth and use of the sense organs, the memory and reason, and ability to speak with accuracy. The vital spirits are also continuing to build themselves and become more and more the actual human self.

The renewal of the teeth and the growing of the hair are manifestations of the superabundance and good condition of kidney *qi*. There is enough kidney *qi* to continue the mental and physical growth, and there is even enough so that internally the preparation for something else is already at work. The result of this process will appear seven years later, at two times seven years old.

Fourteen years old

'At two times seven years fertility arrives.'

Fertility is *tian gui* (天癸). *Tian* (天) is heaven, nature, the natural order, and the power given at the beginning to start a process or a life. It is the power to give the impulse towards manifestation and to determine the specifics of that manifestation. *Gui* (癸) is the tenth of the ten heavenly stems which represents the *yin* of the *yin*, the *yin* of the winter, and the *yin* of the north. The ninth stem is *ren* (壬) which is part of the character for the *ren mai*. *Ren* and *gui*, the ninth and tenth heavenly stems correspond to the water element, to winter, to the kidneys, the north and everything else which resonates with that. The normal presentation in the heavenly stems is to have the *yang* first with the *yin* afterwards. So with *gui* we have the very depths of the *yin*.

The character *gui* may allude to a son making an offering, for example a libation in which liquid is poured onto the soil. This fits well with the image here of water which is in the depths. *Gui* is sometimes associated with something happening in the hidden, damp, darkness of what is below or underground. For instance, in the middle of winter, the deep and secret fertility of the earth starts the process of life which will then appear in springtime. In the Book of Rites it says that tigers mate in the middle of winter. A tiger is a potent symbol of the vital spirits, *jing shen* (精神), and of the vitality based on a perfect *yin yang* balance. If tigers mate in the heart of the winter it is because this is the time for these meetings in the depths to prepare the coming of something which appears in the spring.

Gui (癸) is connected with all these aspects. In the secret heart of the winter the water is not visible because it is not the right season. There is no real rain in the winter because there is no water in heaven, and on earth the water is either frozen or flowing only deep inside the earth. *Gui* therefore implies something in the depths of the earth and linked with water. With the character *tian*, the association is with heaven and the *yang* of heaven, as opposed to the *yin* of water and earth which relate to *gui*. Heaven is also the *yang* associated with the beginning of a process, with the impulse to start given to something. The rich liquids are able to be fertilized because heaven is present.

This expression, *tian gui*, therefore means fertility, because in the liquids of the body there is an impulse coming from heaven which is needed to make life. *Tian gui* is used quite widely to refer to a woman, but it is also used for a man. For example in Suwen chapter 1 the same expression is used for a boy of two times eight years referring to when his fertility and ability to procreate arrives. So this is not only used for women, even if it seems so in later texts. Sometimes it is translated as 'heavenly water', which is not completely wrong, but does not give the whole idea which was in the mind of the Chinese.

What is absolutely clear in *tian gui* is that there is a double expression of heaven and earth, *yin* and *yang*. In the body of a woman the effect will be in the blood and the fertility inside that blood, while the exterior sign will be menstruation. Sometimes another interpretation can be that this character *tian* stands for heavenly authenticity. It implies all the natural authenticity of life which is understood as coming from heaven, even if it is heaven inside. In this context, heaven may represent the whole expression of what was in the original nature of the woman, including the coming of menstruation at the proper time.

At fourteen years old the appropriate stage of development for a girl is to become a woman. The kidney *qi* is able to support the superabundance of its functioning and the production of vital forces. Therefore there is enough blood and *qi* not only to maintain the girl's own life but also to nourish another. So the realization of her authentic, original pattern as a woman is achieved. This is a possible way of looking at the character *tian*, that our natural life is already inside us, and needs only to be followed and accomplished. It is from the inside that this is now possible at fourteen years old. Internally the richness from the *zang* and *fu*, sustained by the kidneys, is able to give *chong* and *ren mai* more to do. The *ren mai* functions fully in so far as previously it was only contributing to growth. Now, at fourteen years old, the superabundance of essences and blood have enough fertility and life for the *ren mai* to offer the uterus a rich blood, and the *chong mai* is able to make this blood circulate, arrive in the uterus and be so full of life that it has the ability to make and sustain a new life.

> '*Ren mai* functions fully while the powerful *chong mai* rises in power.'

The process is imperceptible, but the visible result is that menstruation arrives which is a sign that fresh, good quality blood arrives in the uterus and everything is in the right place with the right movement. The menses flow out regularly because of the mastering of the *chong mai*, while the substance of the blood is offered by the *ren mai*. The kidneys are functioning perfectly, opening and closing and ensuring the richness of the essences, and they allow the liver to operate correctly containing and retaining and then sending forth. The spleen and stomach are also able to make enough blood and *qi* to be used for menstruation and fertility.

Twenty-one years old

> 'At three times seven years the kidney *qi* is even (*ping jun* 平均), then the wisdom teeth grow vigorously.'

This sentence conveys the idea that there is a sort of high point in the functioning of the kidneys, and of the body through the kidneys. Furthermore, the high point is maintained and not declining because there is still a superabundance of *qi* and blood. The strength and the force of life and the kidney *qi* is shown through the wisdom teeth. In Chinese they are called *zhen ya* (真牙). *Zhen* is authentic. Wisdom teeth are the teeth which demonstrate that the authenticity coming from the kidneys is working well and nothing is lost or deficient. The kidneys are therefore able to support the accomplishment of all vital promises. This good and full functioning of the *chong* and *ren mai*, which is also the full functioning of all the organs, is visible externally through the appearance and the vigorous growing of the wisdom teeth. Internally the blood and *qi* make the real fertility of a twenty-one year old woman.

Twenty-eight years old

> 'At four times seven years the muscles and bones are very firm, the hair reaches its greatest length, the body becomes powerful and strong.'

At three times seven years the emphasis was on the *yang* and *qi* with the development of what is firm and hard, for instance the bones and teeth. In a woman of twenty-eight years firmness, strength and power are the main points. These are more *yang* aspects, and show how strong the *yang* of the kidneys is. The accomplishment of that power at four times seven years insists more on the form of the body and the strength realized through the flesh, the muscles and the bones. Here the hair and not the teeth is mentioned. Four is the number appropriate for forms taken on earth, so the woman of twenty-eight realizes all the richness and power of the essences and blood in her body. She has a firmness in her muscles and bones, and a richness in her blood, and this is visible in the growing of her hair until it reaches its greatest length. This is a vigour which exists throughout the whole body at this age.

At twenty-eight a girl is more fleshy which indicates that all the organs are working internally under the sustenance of the kidneys. At three times seven years the kidneys worked for strength, but now at twenty-eight their power is manifest in the whole body form. The blood is rich and the milk is rich. A woman is able to nourish and feed a foetus and child. This is the manifestation of the union between kidneys, liver, spleen and stomach. All of them come together to make the woman's body fluids rich and powerful enough to nourish a child.

Thirty-five years old

Things start to decline at five times seven years:

'At five times seven years the circulations of the *yang ming* decline, the face begins to wrinkle, the hair begins to fall.'

At thirty-five years old there is a natural decline in vitality, something which is also mentioned in Suwen chapter 5, where it states that the *yin* declines by half in a person at forty years old. There is an effervescent power in mid to late teenage when there is an expression of the power in a woman's fertility. After that there is the magnificent strength of the blood and *qi*, which is like a splendour before the harvest. Following that the declines begins. There are signs that there is less superabundance, although a woman is still able to have and nourish children at this age.

We also have to be very careful to remember that in many civilizations, including our own in past times, a woman of thirty-five years old might already be very exhausted by many pregnancies, miscarriages and deliveries, let alone her usual workload. In our current culture a woman of thirty-five will not usually have had many miscarriages or children. She might be exhausted in her kidneys for other reasons such as diet or medication, and if she is exhausted and shows signs of kidney exhaustion it is not very wise for her to have children because she does not have enough strength and enough vitality. If the basis of the kidneys is not strong the relationship with the authentic source of life which enables fertility will be weak. The way in which all the organs work together to produce, maintain and nourish an embryo will also be weak, so in this case it is dangerous, or at least unwise, to start a pregnancy.

What occurs at five times seven years is that the *yang ming* begins to decline and the face begins to wrinkle. This is interesting because the *chong mai* is seen on the face and if there is not enough vitality smooth skin cannot be maintained. The *yang ming* meridian is also on the face and rich in blood and *qi*. If posterior heaven and the spleen and stomach have not renewed enough blood to enrich the *yang ming* because the kidneys are not working as well as they did, there is a decline in the superabundance of blood. The reason this is seen specifically on the face is that the skin is thinnest there.

The hair begins to fall out because that too is not as well nourished as it used to be by good quality blood. Hair shows the superabundance of blood and the same superabundance also makes fertility and the power to nourish an embryo. Every detail is very clear. Normal menstruation, fertility and the ability to produce milk become more and more tiring and draining to the woman's own life. Therefore at six times seven years the ability is lost because of this natural decline.

Forty-two years old

> 'At six times seven years, the three *yang mai* begin their decline above, the whole face wrinkles, the hair begins to whiten.'

Here the decline is of the entire *yang* circulation and because the *yang mai* circulate on the face the effect is seen there. They also circulate around the scalp thus also explaining the whitening of the hair due to a lack of nourishment and strength which should be brought by these meridians. More specific diagnosis can be made according to the area where the hair whitens first. It is mainly the bladder and gallbladder which are involved there. On the face the wrinkles multiply. However, if you are a sage you are able to maintain your smooth skin, and the usual visual presentation of the immortals or the daoists is that they have no wrinkles. They are able to maintain a perfect balance of essences and *qi*.

The fact that wrinkles appear is linked to the decreasing support of the sea of blood and *qi*. Anything which appears at the surface is a manifestation of the internal, authentic process of life, and what is life except the original potential realized through specific circumstances. Performed at the highest level, Chinese face reading is concerned with the manifestation of the inner rhythm of life. *Yang qi* originates in the lower abdomen, linked with the kidneys at the origin, and makes the rhythm and design of the skin, the *li* (理). 'Pattern' is a good word to describe this because the pattern of skin or wrinkles is the pattern of a life. The pattern comes from the depths of the natural life and is visible through the wrinkles which are more linked to the decline of the functioning of the organs.

Forty-nine years old

> 'At seven times seven years the *ren mai* is empty and the powerful *chong mai* declines progressively; fertility dries up. Nothing further passes through the way of earth. The body withers and she no longer has children.'

Although it is 'empty' the *ren mai* will continue to ensure good or at least reasonable functioning of the woman for a while. She will not die for many years to come, but the *ren mai* will not function in the sense that it no longer continues to furnish the uterus with blood or the breasts with milk. It is the same thing with the *chong mai*. It no longer has enough blood and *qi* to nourish the uterus as it did previously. Something is definitely lacking.

If nothing further 'passes through the way of earth' it means that there is no further communication and no further circulation of the superabundance of blood to the uterus by the *mai*. Since nothing comes it dries up and no use can be made of the earth's ability to receive the impulse coming from heaven. The body withers and the woman can no longer have a child. The diminishing of the *yin* is the reason for the diminishing of the strength. So at seven times seven years there is the preparation and arrival of menopause. We will see later on what happens at this time and how a woman reaches a new level of balance in her blood and *qi*.

The following paragraph from Suwen chapter 1 comes after the presentation of man's fertility. One or two points are very specific to men, such as the emission of semen and the whitening of sideburns, but the passage is still applicable to a woman.

> 'The kidneys master (*zhu* 主) the water (*shui* 水) and receive the essences (*jing* 精) of the five *zang* and six *fu* to store (*cang* 藏) them. As long as the five *zang* sustain their rise in power (*sheng* 盛), one is able to produce emissions (*xie* 瀉). But when the five *zang* are in decline (*shuai* 衰), muscles and bones become loose and give way. Fertility has come to its end. Thus the hair and

sideburns whiten, the body grows heavy, walking is no longer secure, one no longer has children.'

The ability to nourish another life is based on sustaining the prosperity of the five *zang*, because what comes from the origin and the original impulse gives the kidneys the power to be the foundation for the good working of life.

INFERTILITY

Infertility in women means that something is not working correctly in the process which should result in fertility. Primarily there is likely to be a weakness in the kidneys which are unable to produce sufficient power of *yin* or *yang*, or to ensure a good enough quality of essences. This will be a kidney weakness with either a *yang* or *yin* deficiency predominating. Secondly there is the involvement of the liver. The liver may be unable to store in order to then send forth. Thirdly there may be an inability to manage body fluids correctly, so that the liquids and richness of the abdomen become problematic and create phlegm and damp. Fourthly there may be a disturbance of the blood which is not life-giving because it is not good enough quality or not circulating properly because of a blockage. This can result in blood stasis. Of course there can be a lot more specific circumstances, for instance exhaustion from many miscarriages, or cold and damp in the uterus. But essentially the four first situations are the main causes of infertility.

Emptiness of the kidneys

An emptiness of the kidneys is exactly the opposite condition to the rising power and prosperity of the *qi* of the kidneys as outlined in Suwen chapter 1. The causes may be various. There might be a weak constitution with a basic insufficiency of the kidneys, or there might be exhaustion of the kidneys because of having sexual relationships too early, or sexuality which is not well managed. There may also be deep exhaustion due to lack of rest or lack of appropriate nourishment. All these things directly attack the force of the kidneys and as a consequence they are unable to ensure the full and proper functioning of the *ren mai* and the great power of the *chong mai*. Therefore *ren mai* and *chong mai* will be empty and weak, and as these circulate to the *bao mai* (胞脈) there will be a weakness in the uterus. This results in an inability to gather and keep the essences in order to allow the beginning of gestation.

In a text from the beginning of the 12th century CE it is said that the causes of infertility in a woman are that *chong* and *ren mai* are insufficient and the *qi* of the kidneys is empty and cold. In another text from the first half of the 14th century it says:

> 'When the *yang* and the essences are displayed and when the *yin* and the blood are able to gather and receive, in this case the essences will form a child. The blood gives it form in the uterus and the embryo starts to exist.'

Therefore, when a woman cannot have children it is very often because there is a deficiency in the blood which is not enough to gather the essences. The lack of richness in blood makes the *yin* movement in the uterus unable to gather and receive and keep the man's semen in order to allow the formation of an embryo. The emptiness of the kidney *qi*, manifest in the decline of the essences and the diminishing of the quality and quantity of blood, means that conception and pregnancy are very difficult.

The emptiness of the kidney *qi*, *chong* and *ren mai* means that their circulation cannot warm up and bring the blood to the uterus, so there are irregularities and disruption in menstruation and possible infertility. The kidney *qi* is not sufficient, so there are signs of kidney deficiency such as pain in the lower area of the body and weakness in the legs coming from the marrow and bones which are unable to support the body with firmness and solidity. At the same time there is also disorder in the mind because the kidneys do not sustain the presence of the spirits of the heart very well. Because the kidneys cannot maintain the *yin* and the essences in the head there are symptoms such as dizziness and tinnitus.

We can see more precisely what happens when there is a predominantly *yang* or *yin* deficiency. With a *yang* deficiency very often menstruation comes late with scanty blood of a pale colour. This is because the *yang* of the kidneys is empty, so there is not enough warmth in the lower heater, and not enough dynamism in the circulation coming to the uterus. Cold prevails and invades the whole area. This means that the circulation is deficient and difficult, and the woman cannot become pregnant.

There are also other signs of kidney *yang* deficiency such as pain in the lower part of the abdomen which is where the power of the kidneys is located and is the place where the kidneys themselves are found. It is also on the vertical axis of the body with all the power of the marrow and bones supporting the uprightness of the trunk. The subtle movement of this area needs the *qi* and essences of the kidneys to be in a good state. When there is a deficiency there can be an effect in the interchanges and circulation in that area. Cold, or lack of *yang*, could lead to pain and the inability to walk well. These are exactly the same things we would find with a decline in the fire of *ming men*.

Because of the decline of kidney *yang* and the fire of *ming men* very often there is also an insufficient warming of the spleen and stomach and the whole middle heater. In this case it is said that the fire of *ming men* is unable to warm the *yang* of the spleen. Consequently there is difficulty in transforming and managing damp and there may be soft stools and perhaps even diarrhoea. At the same time, because the *yang* of the kidneys is unable to warm up the lower abdomen and help transform the *qi* and liquids of the bladder, there may be abnormal urination. The urine will be clear, cold and abundant. The kidneys are also unable to transform the essences to make rich marrow, so the marrow cannot give the bones their solidity and strength. This is first perceived in the legs where all the weight of the body is supported. There will be pain, weakness and a lack of strength in the legs.

There may be other signs too, such as cold in the lower abdomen and the possibility of pain there too. There is often a diminishing of the libido, and clear vaginal discharges, sometimes of great quantity. The tongue is normally pale with a white coat, and the pulse is either deep (*chen* 沉) and thin (*xi* 細), deep and slow (*chi* 遲), or deep and weak (*ruo* 弱).

Treatment is geared to tonifying the kidneys and warming up the uterus, while at the same time regulating and supporting the *ren* and *chong mai*. Using acupuncture points there are many options such as Ren 4, Du 4, Kidney 3, Spleen 6, Bladder 23, or Gallbladder 26 which is a point on the *dai mai*. You can also apply moxibustion on *ren mai* to warm up the whole lower abdomen.

With emptiness of the *yin* of the kidneys, the blood and menstruation is scanty. Normally the colour of the blood is darker too, while with emptiness of the *yang* the colour would be pale. With *yin* deficiency the blood is normally without clots. There is a deterioration in the quality of the blood and the essences, and it means an emptiness of the authentic *yin*. Therefore the quality of the essences is not good and they are not enough to generate sufficient good quality blood. The *chong* and *ren mai* are unable to act normally because they do not have the blood they need to function properly. There are therefore consequences at several levels.

The insufficiency of blood and essences leads to symptoms where the pure essences should work, for instance the upper orifices and specifically the eyes and ears. The ears are linked with the kidney essences of course, and with a deficiency there may be vertigo and dizziness. At the same time if the kidney essences are not nourishing the heart there may be heart palpitations and difficulty in sleeping. There can also be pain and weakness in the legs. Due to the emptiness of *yin* there is often the development of inner heat. The quantity of blood diminishes, there may be heat in the five hearts (palms, soles of feet, chest), and possible menstrual irregularities. Normally the tongue is red with little coating, and the pulse is deep and thin. If the inner heat develops a lot, then the pulse may be fast and thin. However, there is no force because of the emptiness of the *yin*. There is also the possibility of weakness or pain in the knees.

The treatment is to nourish the kidneys and maintain the blood in order to regulate all the functions of *chong* and *ren mai*. If the signs of inner heat are very strong and there is fever, you need to clear heat, calm the fire and nourish and irrigate the authentic *yin*. This situation can also lead to an obstruction of the liver *qi*, in which case the treatment needs adapting in anther way.

Obstruction of the liver

Very often obstruction of the liver is due to emotions and the inability to make the heart *qi* circulate well enough to resolve the concerns. There are many potential causes of this kind of situation. For instance, there may be worries coming from the spleen blocking the movement of the liver. Or within the liver itself there can be excitement and resentment without the possibility of expression so that they become suppressed anger. There can be suspicion and jealousy which cannot be spoken openly. In fact with the liver there are many possibilities of not being able to free oneself of a feeling which is gnawing away inside. This is the difference between obstruction of the liver and obstruction of the spleen: the liver has the feeling of being blocked inside and unable to work properly or free the circulation as it should, and therefore there is a lack of harmony between blood and *qi* in the liver. In some texts this is called an inability of the *chong* and *ren mai* to cooperate and the result is that we do not have the necessary richness for the beginning of an embryo.

If we look at a text from the beginning of the 19th century, the Zhuangqingzhunüke, a gynecological treatise, published in 1827, there is a discussion about a woman who cannot conceive because her liver *qi* are obstructed and knotted. The main consequence of this blockage is the inability of the liver to spread out and make things circulate throughout the body. The rhythm of storing and delivering on time is disturbed, so menstruation is irregular, being sometimes late and sometimes early. Very often when it does come the abdomen is painful because the circulation is blocked. Because of the liver's difficulty in making things circulate properly it is also hard for the blood to circulate to the uterus, so the blood is dark and possibly clotted. The quantity of blood will also be irregular, sometimes scanty and sometimes abundant. Circulation in the liver meridian is where the *qi* express themselves, so particularly before menstruation when everything is more congested and blocked, there may be pain and swelling in the breasts. There is also the possibility of pain and swelling in the whole chest and rib area.

Because of the obstruction of the liver *qi* there may also be an instability psychologically. A woman may become very irritatable, or agitated and easily angered. Or there may be a blockage of the *qi* which leads instead to a sense of oppression, with deep sighing in order to try and free the blockage. Normally the tongue is red with a thin coat and the pulse is wiry (*xian* 弦).

The treatment given is to relax the liver, re-establish the circulation and to reorganize the working of the *chong* and *ren mai*. You have to be very careful with the specific details of the woman's presentation. For instance, sweat and congestion of the chest and ribs are very significant, or if there is swelling in the breasts even up to the point of clots and masses. Or whether the swelling in the breast comes with heat and acute pain. If the obstruction of the liver leads to a great agitation in the woman's psychological state, with a lot of dreams and agitated sleep, then the treatment has to be modified another way. With acupuncture local points such as Stomach 29, and points on the liver meridian such as Liver 3 may be used. Spleen 6 is also useful, and you may use points such as Large Intestine 4 to unblock the circulation and stasis. For congestion in the chest you could use Heart Master 6. You can also use local points on the *ren mai*, for instance Ren 3.

Phlegm and damp

Very often infertility due to phlegm and damp is found in women who are overweight. This can be due to a diet too rich in fat or to an accumulation of phlegm and damp. Phlegm and damp make circulation and movement of *qi* difficult which leads to blockage which can also occur at the level of the uterus. This hampers the circulations going to the uterus: *bao luo* (胞絡) and *bao mai* (胞脈). There is no possibility that the blood can be well nourished and rich in essences, so the process of gestation cannot start. In the same text from the 19th century, the Zhuangqingzhunüke, it says that there is infertility from phlegm and obesity when the woman is fat and the phlegm and liquids are abundant inside the body, so that she is unable to conceive.

With phlegm and damp there is an inability of the clear to rise up and govern the turbid, so in this situation there would be other signs of the lack of circulation and the failure of the clear *yang* to rise up such as dizziness, palpitations, congestion in the chest and even vomiting. If the spleen is completely congested by damp it is unable to transport and transform the fluids. Consequently, turbid liquids descend in the abdomen causing vaginal discharges which are abundant and thick. The main aim for treatment is to dry the damp and transform the phlegm. This allows the blood to circulate in the uterus again normally.

Symptoms in the heart must be considered too. Heart palpitations need calming. If menstruation stops or is even just late you need to see if the kidneys are weak and cold. In this case treatment would also need to warm up the kidneys. Using acupuncture there are many possibilities for treatment. With phlegm and damp obstructing the circulation it means you need to work on the liver in order to open the pathways of the *qi* circulation and get rid of the blockage, using points such as Ren 4, Ren 6, Spleen 6, Liver 3, Bladder 20, or even Bladder 31 to open circulation in the specific area. If there is cold and damp in the uterus you may need to use Du 4, with moxibustion too if the cold is very intense. Ren 4, Ren 3, Ren 8, Ren 6 and Stomach 29 are also useful. If the cold and damp have completely blocked the uterus then you can use Ren 5 and Spleen 9, and Stomach 28 as well.

Blood stasis

Sometimes having sexual relationships during menstruation is given as a reason for blood stasis in gynaecological texts. There is also the possibility of cold in the uterus blocking the blood and causing stagnation. There is a quotation from a book from the first half of the 18th century which says that it is because blood has remained accumulated in the uterus that new blood cannot enter in and start an embryo. The retained blood injures the functioning of *chong* and *ren mai* and stops the process of conception. If these do not work properly it will result in blockage, and the lack of circulation of the *chong* and *ren mai* means there is a weakness in the uterus's circulation. The blood cannot be regularly renewed and cannot make what blood there is fertile. Because of the stasis menstruation may be late and scanty, with the possibility of clots and pain in the lower abdomen. Quite often the menstrual blood is also very dark, and the stasis causes intense pain in the lower abdomen which the woman does not want touched.

When the *qi* is weak and lacking the blood stasis in the uterus is not moved by the circulation so there can be other disturbances in the blood. If *chong* and *ren mai* are weak there will often be spotting or continuous bleeding from the uterus. Other parts of the body can also show the effect of blood stasis. For example, it is possible to have an effect visible on the skin because the blood is unable to nourish it and so it loses its smoothness and becomes rough. You can also observe signs of blood stasis under the eyes where it will show dark. The pulse is deep and, according to particular circumstances, it can be deep and thin or deep and stringy.

Treatment is aimed at making the blood circulate normally and removing the stasis by transforming it through the effect of *qi*. Often it is necessary to warm up and re-establish the circulation since the *qi* and the *yang* make the circulation of the blood warm within the uterus. However, you must be very careful if there are signs of a blocked liver which can arise as a consequence of blood stasis. If a woman has had many miscarriages this can lead to an insufficiency of kidney *qi*, or the miscarriage itself may be due to kidney *qi* insufficiency. In this case the best help is to treat before another pregnancy. With acupuncture you can use points such as Kidney 3, Bladder 33, Du 20, Spleen 6, Stomach 36 and Bladder 17, which are recommended for infertility due to frequent miscarriages.

MENOPAUSE

As we saw in Suwen chapter 1 menopause is not a disease. However, in the body of a woman difficulties may arise because from five times seven years her fertility begins to decline. At a certain age, around forty-nine to fifty years old, there is a turning point for a woman after which there is no longer enough richness and strength to form an embryo. So the menopause is the name given to all the changes arising in the body of a woman which are the consequence of the weakening power of the kidneys. There is weakness in the *yin*, and everywhere in the woman's body the diminishing of the *yin* root of life means that the movement and transformation of the *qi* and *yang*, which allow the work and gathering of the essences, is undermined. Therefore the quantity of blood is no longer enough and at the same time there is the danger of an imbalance between the blood and *qi*, *yin* and *yang*. This can be especially so in the liver thereby creating fire of the liver or a counter current of the *qi* due to the weakness of the *yin* and the insufficiency of the blood. Sometimes, depending on the constitution of the woman, there is the possibility of weakness in the *yang* and a subsequent lack of *qi*. In this case there will be other symptoms and characteristics during the menopause. In either case, it is primarily and fundamentally at the level of the kidneys that the changes occur.

At this point a woman has to change to another model of life which is not obviously one of richness and superabundance. She has to achieve a new organization of life within her, having what is plentiful enough just for her alone. This is easier for her to do if she does not feel the lack or loss of something. If she is calm and quiet and without excessive emotions and desires about it she will be able to accept and enjoy this new period of her life. Very often there are problems linked with the investments she has made in her life and the value she has placed on them. If she believes her worth as a woman is based on the potential of the superabundance and the richness, one way or another she will be in trouble when that superabundance is no longer able to sustain her goal or purpose. This is something which we find constantly in the clinic.

During the menopause a woman is in danger of the water being less able to contain the fire, and the kidneys to keep the root. The weakness of the kidneys is related to the diminishing and emptiness of the *yin*. This results in too great a power of the liver which can deteriorate into irritation and anger, resentment and so on. These feelings are common for a woman at this time of life to experience. This aggravates the state of balance between blood and *qi*.

This is also a time when the kidneys and heart have difficulty in communicating and balancing each other so it is more difficult to keep a calm mind. This is due to the weakness of the kidney essences. A woman must try to overcome these situations and imbalances, and keep an even state throughout the difficulties associated with the diminishing of the *yin* and the weakening of the *yang*. She must try not to excite the *qi* any more or increase the disorder in the blood.

Menopause is a stage of life in which a woman ought to be able to be calm and serene and not overworked, or tired and exhausted. Exhaustion will only aggravate the situation in the liver, spleen and kidneys. She needs to be at peace in her life and in herself and her relationships. But if we look at the situation of most women arriving at their late forties these days there are two possibilities. Either she is at the top of her career with a lot of responsibility and accompanying stress, or she has already lost her job and is unable to find another one because she is too old! At that age she has very often started to take care of elderly parents, which is a process that may last for years. Perhaps she still takes care of her own children, who although grown up are not completely out of the house. Or if they are out of the house then maybe she has started to take care of the grandchildren. It is also a period during which her husband is probably around fifty as well and she has to keep an eye on him! In the middle of all this the poor woman must not worry, be exhausted or get irritable!

All this is very different from the situation in past centuries with women reaching forty years old exhausted by multiple pregnancies, deliveries and miscarriages. But there are still a lot of reasons for contemporary women to be exhausted at this stage of life. Usually we see the effects of the diminishing strength of the kidneys, as described in Suwen chapter 1:

'As long as the five *zang* sustain their rise in power one is able to produce emissions. But when the five *zang* are in decline, muscles and bones become loose and give way. Fertility has come to its end. Thus the hair and sideburns whiten, the body grows heavy, walking is no longer secure, one no longer has children.'

As usual we must make a distinction between the weakening of the *yin* or the *yang* of the kidneys. Particularly during menopause, there is an interaction between both with a changing imbalance between the *yin* and *yang*. First you have the strengthening of one and the weakening of the other, but then very often after a while both decline together in various disorders. Quite often some of the signs of disturbance during the menopause are similar to what occurs before and during menstruation, due to the same reason which is the increasing emptiness of the blood of the liver on one side and of the *yin* of the kidneys on the other. We also often see the consequences of the rising *yang* of the liver or the fire of the heart.

Kidney yin deficiency

With weakness of the kidney *yin* there are often clinical signs such as dizziness, vertigo and tinnitus, because the kidney essences are no longer able to irrigate and nourish the upper orifices and the brain, and specifically the ear. Also there is often agitation during sleep with a lot of dreams, or difficulty in sleeping and insomnia. These symptoms come from the deterioration of the essences and the diminishing of the blood, so that it is no longer able to keep the *hun* (魂) in their dwelling place in the liver. Disturbed dreams result and there is agitation, heat and uneasiness in the area of the heart. There is a loss of what nourishes and maintains the heart. This also results in insomnia, agitation, palpitations, and the lack of nourishment for the liver and heart promotes irritability, fever and hot flushes. In the clinic you must always look at the timing and quantity of these hot flushes, and whether they come with other symptoms.

There is also the possibility of redness or flushing in the face, specifically in the area of the cheekbones which reflect the kidneys. Dryness in the mouth, but without any desire to drink, occurs as a result of the lack of liquids and the diminishing of the kidney *yin*. There are several levels of dryness and thirst which relate to the degree of weakness of the *yin* and the resulting fire inside the body. With reactive fire there can also be heat in what are called the five hearts, or there may be actual fever. The dryness may show in constipation. There may be daytime sweating or night sweats because of the emptiness of the *yin*, the inner fire and the force of the *yang* being too great. Weakness and pain might also be seen in the lower area of the knees.

Other signs of deterioration are also possible, for example if the fire of the heart is not restrained there may be strong cardiac palpitations, loss of memory and even mental disturbance. If the *yang* of the liver rises up too strongly due to the lack of kidney *yin* then there may be vertigo, dizziness or headaches. In these cases treatment has to balance the liver and calm the inner wind. Sometimes heat enters the blood, if this happens at the same time as wind is created, it causes itching in the skin or the feeling that ants are walking on the skin or in the flesh.

In treatment it is always possible to try to nourish and sustain the liver and kidneys with points such as Bladder 23, Bladder 18, Kidney 3, Spleen 6, or Spleen 10 for the blood, and Liver 2 to help clear liver fire. It is a question of regulating the *qi* and maintaining a good movement of liver and kidney *qi*. A point such as Kidney 3 may be used to sustain the water of the kidneys and to help struggle against heat due to the emptiness of *yin*. Liver 2 and Spleen 10 may be needled together to regulate the *qi* and the blood, and Spleen 6 is always useful.

If the force of the *yang* leads to agitation and fire of the heart, also visible in the small intestine and the bladder as damp urination, you can use Heart Master 7 to calm the heart and the spirits of the mind. You can also treat and balance the heart by using points such as Bladder 15 and Heart 7.

Kidney yang deficiency

If weakness of the *yin* and reactive inner heat evolve into a situation of exhaustion and lack of *yang* and circulation, the symptoms will change. There may be blockage of the liver *qi* by depression and despondency. This can occur in a menopause which starts with a deficiency of kidney *yang*. In this case there will not be agitation and irritability but rather depression, despondency and oppression, with a lack of reaction and apathy. There will also be other signs of the decline of the fire of *ming men* and *yang* in the body such as a general cooling and sensitivity to the cold, and specifically with cold in the hands and feet. There will be an effect on the body liquids as well because the *yang qi* is less and less able to work on the water or to sustain the *yang* of the spleen to work on the damp and liquids. The result is that body fluids are not well transformed and transported and so there may be oedema in the legs or perhaps even in the face. At the same time there are liquid stools, which are another sign of the inability of the kidney *yang* to warm up the *yang* of the spleen.

An emptiness of the *yang* of the kidneys is sometimes part of what is called the double emptiness of the *yang* of the kidneys and spleen. In this situation treatment should sustain, warm up and tonify both the kidneys and spleen. Bladder 20 and 23, the back *shu* points, are both used for this. Bladder 20 may also be used with Spleen 6 in order to regulate the *qi* of the spleen. Because the *qi* of the spleen are able to contain the blood in the right place the blood circulates in the correct places and the *qi*, being renewed wisely, can improve all the circulation.

Bladder 23 and Ren 4 can be used to work on the relationship with the origin, to strengthen the root and give the best possible power to the *qi* coming from the kidneys. Ren 6, the sea of *qi*, also works on the relationship with the origin, and enables the *qi* to follow nature and the natural order. When the *qi* are in the right place and are the right strength, the blood will follow and proper nourishment of the liver and the kidneys will be re-established. You can also use points such as Du 4 to tonify the authentic *yang* and dissipate all the damp and stagnation which was due to the lack of *yang*.

With the heart, when the fire is out of control and no longer balanced by the water of the kidneys, there will be symptoms such as palpitations, insomnia, excessive dreaming and perhaps even confusion and mental disturbance. In this situation treatment must nourish the kidneys and stabilize the heart.

MENSTRUAL PROBLEMS

Commentaries on the Neijing Suwen chapter 7 tell us that disturbance of menstruation and amenorrhoea are due to three main causes. First is an emptiness of the spleen and stomach, second is a dysfunction of the *ren* and *chong mai*, and third is a blockage due to phlegm and damp. In chapter 7 the problem is linked with a weakness of the spleen and stomach, because if these are not functioning, for physical or psychological reasons such as worry or obsession, there is a lack of harmony between the spleen and the heart which results in an inability to assimilate nutriments and maintain circulation. This is a situation where the blood diminishes day after day until the situation reaches what is referred to as dryness of the blood. Dryness of the blood is a kind of amenorrhoea in which there is no possibility of any menstrual flow let alone conception. Dryness of the blood is described in Suwen chapter 40:

'The Emperor said: "What is this kind of disease where there is a pressure and a congestion in the chest and rib area leading to an impossibility to eat. It is as if there is an obstacle in swallowing the food. When the disease develops fully and is not just an unease, there is first a rancid and raw meat smell, and clear liquids are expelled from the mouth. There is spitting of blood. The four limbs are cold and there is dizziness, and sometimes there is bleeding from the two lower orifices. What is this kind of disease?"

Qi Bo replied: "The name of this disease is dryness of the blood (*xue ku* 血枯). One gets this disease by suffering a great loss of blood in youth, or by having sexual relationships when drunk. The *qi* diminish and the liver is injured, causing the menses gradually to stop coming.'"

A blockage or difficulty in circulation of the *qi* means the blood cannot circulate. This may come from psychological reasons, for instance involving blockage of the liver *qi* by suppressed anger or jealousy. An erratic and irregular circulation of the blood arises due to this blockage of the liver, something which in later books is called a disharmony and deficiency in the functioning of the *chong* and *ren mai*. It is an injury made to the sea of blood, or to the way the *qi* manage the blood in the sea of blood. There may be haemorrhages and irregular menstruation. Phlegm and damp also block the circulation which brings the blood to nourish and irrigate the uterus, so there is a blockage of the sea of blood which leads to disturbance in menstruation, with late menstruation, amenorrhoea, or a lot of turbid liquids present in the abdomen.

This disease is due to a severe lack of blood. The lack of blood damages the liver because it can no longer rely on having or storing good quality blood. Because of the diminishing blood and the weakness of the *yin*, in the end there is a drying up of the *qi* due to the fact that the *qi* are renewed from the essences and blood. It is the reason why the text speaks also of an injury on the liver *qi* and not just of a dryness of the blood.

The pressure and congestion in the chest and rib area relate to the lung and the liver respectively. Normally the liver stores the blood and the lung masters the *qi*. When everything is normal the *qi* are able to move and make the blood circulate properly, but if there is a weakness and deficiency of blood then the *qi* are unable to direct and guide the blood properly. This creates a counter current in the *qi* of the lung and liver which explains the congestion and feeling of pressure in the ribs and chest. The feeling of blockage is also felt at the throat, and causes an obstacle to swallowing. The blockage and counter current of the liver *qi* generate heat which also, due to the counter current and blockage of *qi* of the lung, burns up the liquids in the lung and prevents the descending movement of the lung being carried out properly. The blockage of *qi* explains the smells which are associated with the liver and lung respectively, rancid and raw meat.

If there is a congestion of the liver *qi* then there is a blockage in the circulation. In this situation the spleen is damaged and cannot assure proper transformation and transportation. Damp and liquids are not transformed correctly and damp and turbid damp invade the stomach so that it cannot make anything descend. Therefore clear liquids come out of the mouth. There is also inner heat due to the blockage of the lung *qi* which puts pressure on the capillaries and explains the spitting of blood. When there is such an obstruction that the liver and lung *qi* are blocked then the spleen and stomach damp becomes more important, and the clear *yang* coming from the work of the spleen and stomach cannot be spread to warm the four limbs, so there is a lack of renewal of the defensive *qi*, disturbance of the chest and lung, with the result that the four limbs cool down.

There are also other possible symptoms on the pathway of the liver *qi*. The liver meridian connects with the head and eyes on its way to the vertex. In the case of insufficiency of liver *yin*, which is the situation here because of the lack of blood, the liver *yang* will rise up too impetuously resulting in problems with the eyes and vision. The rising *yang* is an agitation reflecting the lack of *yin* and blood, and it disturbs the areas where the liver *qi* and meridian penetrate, so there are dizziness, vertigo and disturbed vision. Obstruction of the liver may also generate a heat which disturbs normal circulation or gathering of blood in the lower heater. In this instance there may be blood which is forced out through the lower orifices by the heat coming from the blocked liver.

There are very few herbal formulas mentioned in the Suwen but one is given for this condition. Qi Bo tells the Emperor that you can treat this condition using cuttle fish. The nature of cuttle fish is salty and gently warming, and it is a very good ingredient to use for leakages, for vaginal discharges and amenorrhoea, and drying up of the blood. It is said that cuttle fish is good for all women's diseases, specifically where the liver is damaged and there is blood leaking from the lower orifices.

Amenorrhoea

Amenorrhoea can be presented in two ways. First one can say that there are two kinds of amenorrhoea: *xue ku* (血 枯), dryness of blood, which we have just examined in looking at Suwen chapter 40, and blood stasis (*xue zhi* 血 滯). We can make a clear differentiation between them.

Dryness of the blood *xue ku* 血 枯

In the case of dryness of the blood there will have been a large loss of blood for one reason or another. The cause may be exhausting sexual relationships, multiple pregnancies, deliveries or miscarriages, or a long illness. Emotional worries and concerns can also dry up the blood, as can general tiredness. All of these weaken the production of blood by the spleen and stomach. They become unable to produce and renew blood normally, so there is a diminishing at the very source of the regeneration of the *yin* of the blood. As a consequence the liver is not well nourished with sufficient blood, and there may also be a more severe injury to the kidneys resulting in their weakness.

The drying up of the sources of the *yin* and the blood results in a reduction or cessation of menstruation. Usually there are accompanying symptoms of emptiness, for instance disturbance in digestion, an inability to taste food, a decrease in appetite, or semi-liquid stools. The diminishing *yin* causes a lack of irrigation and smoothness which is visible at the lips and the nails which relate to the spleen and liver respectively. The complexion is often yellowish and all the skin can be rough and dry. There may also be weight loss due to the dryness of blood leading to a lack of nutrition of the flesh. The lack of essences will also lead to a lack of vital spirits.

Treatment aims to sustain the *yin* using points such as Bladder 17, which is the *hui* (會) point of the blood, and Bladder 20 for the spleen, or even Bladder 18, the *shu* (輸) point of the liver. These three points nourish the spleen and liver, but often you also have to sustain and nourish the kidneys. The source of the blood needs taking care of via the spleen and stomach using points such as Stomach 36 and Spleen 6 to reinforce the source of blood and *qi* renewal. Points on the *ren mai* can be used in order to help the circulation of blood and *qi* and to harmonize them. Ren 4 and Ren 6 are good for this. If you want to work on the spleen and stomach you can also use Stomach 36 with Bladder 20, or in the case of anaemia Spleen 10 with Bladder 17 (*shu* (輸) point of the diaphragm and *hui* (會) point of the blood). Points such as Ren 5 and Stomach 25, which is the *mu* point of the large intestines on the Stomach meridian, regulate all transportation. For semi-liquid stools you can use Bladder 25 and Stomach 25. The *mu* point of the triple heater, Ren 5, can also be helpful. For the other symptoms such as dizziness and palpitations you need to add relevant points such as Du 20 and Heart Master 6.

Blood stasis *xue zhi* 血滯

Blood stasis often has an origin in the person's psychological state and the seven emotions, specifically in obsessive worries or oppression. Resentment and anger can also be responsible. Obstruction of the liver *qi* blocks the free circulation of blood and leads to blood stasis. Another main cause may be cold. Cold might seem to be a sign of *yang* deficiency but there is also cold which enters the uterus, perhaps because of drinking very cold drinks during menstruation. The cold blocks circulation in the lower abdomen creating symptoms which at first seem to be of fullness.

Menstruation stops sooner with blood stasis than with dryness of blood. The lower abdomen is painful and is made worse by touch. The pain is continuous, not intermittent, and there can be swelling of the abdomen with the possibility of fever and agitation. Painful clots or masses can form in the abdomen, and there is the possibility of constipation or dry, dark black stools. Treatment must break up the stasis, deal with the inner heat and stimulate the circulation of the blood. Work should be carried out mainly on the liver, spleen and *ren mai*, mainly dispersing.

On the liver meridian coupling the water point, Liver 8, and the fire point, Liver 2, helps the circulation of *qi* in the meridian, easing congestion, breaking blockages and regulating the flow of liver *qi*. On the *ren mai*, Ren 3 is a meeting with the liver meridian, the *jue yin* of the foot. Therefore it can be chosen to regulate the lower heater and to work on *ren mai*, *chong mai* and liver *qi*. A point such as the *xi* cleft point of the spleen meridian, Spleen 8, is also good, as is the emerging point of the *chong mai*, Stomach 30. These give an impulse to all the circulation guiding the blood.

Spleen 6 and Large Intestine 4 are also useful in unblocking the circulation. Large Intestine 4 is very good in cases of blockage and congestion due to heat in the *qi*. Spleen 6 is better for blockage and stasis of the blood. Needling both together means you can free the circulation of blood and *qi*. Local points such as Stomach 29 and Bladder 32 are also helpful to open up and re-establish circulation linked to the uterus. Spleen 10 is always good for the movement of the blood, and can be used with Liver 2 to free up the liver circulation and regulate the spleen, and as a result to slowly diminish the heat and promote circulation. For oppression in the thorax area with heat and agitation you can use Heart Master 6 and Kidney 6, which is also a point of the *yin qiao mai*.

As mentioned before there is also another approach in differentiating amenorrhoea. You can still determine if there is dryness of blood or blood stasis, emptiness or fullness, but you can also focus on the organ functions to be more precise. Therefore there may be situations where there is emptiness and weakness of blood and *qi* but also weakness and insufficiency of the liver and kidneys. These are not exactly the same thing. There may be emptiness of *yin* and dryness of blood, but there may be blood stagnation or blockage due to phlegm and damp as well, and understanding these differences allows the treatment to focus more accurately.

Liver and kidney deficiency

Amenorrhoea due to a deficiency of the kidneys and a resulting deficiency of the liver, is usually caused by problems in the constitution itself, or where a woman had a lot of health problems when she was very young. As a result her fertility, the *tian gui*, did not arrive. The strength of her kidneys, by means of which the liquids are enriched with the power to make life, is too impaired. Or there may have been an early marriage or sexual experience, or many pregnancies and deliveries which damaged the liver and kidneys and led to the deterioration of the essences and the diminution of the blood. In this case *chong* and *ren mai* have lost what should ensure their maintenance. This is all stated in a gynaecological textbook from the beginning of the 13th century CE (the Furen daquanliangfang):

'When the *qi* of the kidneys is fully prosperous *chong* and *ren mai* circulate and flow nicely and the blood of menstruation is abundant and descends timely. If not, there is no circulation.'

Another text from the Yixue zhengzhuan, by Yu Tuan, published in 1515 says:

'Menstruation depends on the distribution and transformation of the water of the kidneys. If the water of the kidneys has deteriorated then the menstrual blood dries up.'

In this situation something is wrong with the development of the woman, and this might be the case with a young woman of eighteen or so who has not yet started menstruating. Or perhaps there is menstruation but it is scanty and pale and irregular. It means that the development of the kidneys, which make fertility possible, has been incomplete or imperfect. As a result nothing is offered to the liver to store and release, so the sea of blood cannot work properly. In this case there would normally be other signs of the kidney deficiency at the same time, for instance dizziness, tinnitus, or pain and lack of strength in the lower legs or knees coming from the bones and marrow. Usually the tongue is pale with little coating, and the pulse deep and weak, or thin and circulating with difficulty. This situation needs treatment which focuses on tonification of the kidneys and nourishing of the liver.

Emptiness of blood and *qi*

Amenorrhoea in this case is not linked with the constitution and the way in which fertility and the mechanism of menstruation evolves. Here the woman has no specific problems with her constitution or problems in the early stages of her life, but for some reason there has been an injury to the spleen which also touches the heart. This could be due to a very poor diet or exhaustion, or to an error in treatment for example. With Chinese medicine, if a therapist made a mistake in diagnosis or the dosage of herbs, the woman might suffer a great loss of vitality from sweating or purging. This would affect the spleen and pass from the spleen to the heart. The *qi* of the spleen and the source of the renewal of blood and *qi* is diminished, and as a result an injury is inflicted on the heart which is not nourished properly. This is a situation which we find explained in a gynaecological textbook from the beginning of the 19th century, the Yeshinüke zhengzhi, attributed to Ye Gui, and published in 1817:

> 'The heart is the master of *qi* and blood, and the spleen is the foundation of *qi* and blood. If worries and concerns injure the heart the *qi* of the heart is empty and deteriorated. It is no longer able to generate the blood. The spleen is the son of the heart, as a consequence the spleen loses what maintains and nourishes it. Therefore there is no desire to eat and drink. As a result

there is an interruption in the source of all the transformations maintaining life.'

Very often in this situation menstruation is late and scanty, and gradually this evolves into amenorrhoea because of the diminution of the quantity of blood at the very source of the heart and spleen. The colour of the blood is pale. There is a lack of harmony and balance between the blood and *qi* of the heart because of this insufficiency. The descending movement is reduced and the *qi* is not stabilized by the *yin* and blood, so it sometimes results in palpitations. At the same time, because of the lack of nourishment to the heart, there may be a mental tiredness, and the woman's complexion will show the lack of blood and be pale. The blood is insufficient to make the skin and flesh flourish.

Since the spleen is empty, the *yang* of the middle heater cannot support the *qi* in general or the specific *qi* of the upper heater, chest and lung. This will have an effect on the *qi* of the sea of *qi* in the middle of the chest, the ancestral *qi* also called the gathering *qi* (*zong qi* 宗氣) because the *qi* coming from nutrition is not enough to renew these *qi*. Therefore there is a lack of *qi* in the chest and shortness of breath with slowness in speaking since there is no strength there either. The woman will have difficulty in speaking because of the lung *qi*'s lack of power. Normally the tongue coat is white and the pulse is deep and weak. The aim of treatment is to increase the *qi* and tonify the blood.

If the heart palpitations are strong or her mental state

is poor, these are also important factors. Or if there is a deficiency of essences and blood in the kidneys, or a weakness of the *qi* and essences of the kidneys, perhaps if the woman has lost a lot of blood and *qi* after delivery, then these things must be considered too. Body and armpit hair are good areas to assess the state of the blood and *qi*, and whether her hair falls out. Dryness of the vagina and lack of libido are also good indicators of the level of deficiency in essences and blood or the level of weakness of the kidneys *qi*.

Emptiness of *yin*

This is a situation in which the *yin* and the blood dry up due to the state of the constitution, or because of a chronic emptiness of blood. The effects of medication may also dry up the *yin* of the kidneys. This is very close to the condition we saw described in Suwen chapter 40. The *yin*, the nutrition and the essences deteriorate and there is internal reactive fire burning up the body fluids and leading to an even greater drying up of the *yin* and blood. This then causes amenorrhoea. In the chapter on gynaecology in his complete works, published in 1624, Zhang ziebin said that with dryness of the *yin* and dryness of the blood there may be amenorrhoea with coughing and night fever. This is therefore emptiness of *yin* with inner heat as a consequence.

Normally dryness of blood and body fluids is explained by the diminution of the blood and by the effect of the fire and the floating *yang*, because the *yang* cannot be kept inside by the richness of the *yin* and blood. There are symptoms of agitation and uneasiness in the chest, heat in the centre of the feet and palms (the heat of the five hearts), fever with sweating, hot flushes with whiteness of the cheekbones, and also injury to the lung capillaries leading to a cough with spitting of blood. Normally the tongue is red with little coating and the pulse is stringy, wiry and fast. If the inner fire is not strong there may be a thin and imperceptible pulse.

What needs to be done in treatment is to maintain and nourish the *yin* and at the same to clarify the heat. The treatment needs to be tailored to the intensity and characteristics of the inner heat. For instance, if the fever is strong or if there is more activity in the lung with coughing and spitting of blood, or if the symptoms come more from the heart with insomnia or cardiac palpitations, then different points need to be added. Likewise if there is dryness of the blood and the burning up of all liquids, even to the point of what we call tuberculosis.

Blockage of *qi* and blood stasis

Amenorrhoea is often due to emotional causes causing an obstruction in the liver *qi* and preventing the circulation of blood to the uterus, or by a blockage due to cold preventing the circulation from flowing normally. This is found described in the Wanshinüke, published in 1549 by Wan Quan, a great gynaecologist of the 16th century who said:

'Oppressing griefs, worries and concerns cause the *qi* to be blocked, then the blood is congested and menstruation no longer arrives.'

Because there is a blockage in the circulation there is pain and distension, particularly in the lower abdomen. There can be swelling in the rib area too, which is another manifestation of the blockage of *qi*. The *qi* are unable to make the blood circulate, and *chong mai* and *ren mai* can no longer ensure free circulation and normal communication with the uterus, so menstruation does not occur. The emotions and mind are also blocked, so the liver may be irritable at the same time as there is all the congestion in the ribs and lower abdomen.

The main focus of treatment here is to restore the blood circulation and dissolve the stasis in order to restore a normal movement of the *qi* and re-establish menstruation. Normally the tongue would be dark with red maculae showing the stasis. The pulse would be deep, wiry and stringy.

Phlegm and damp

Amenorrhoea from phlegm and damp occurs in a woman who is corpulent or obese, or who has a weakness in her *yang* and *qi*. Because of the weakness damp and liquids cannot be transformed and transported, so they accumulate in the woman's body, move downwards and block the proper functioning of the *chong* and *ren mai* and the circulation bringing blood to the uterus.

The blood expresses what is called the water of the kidneys, or the essences of life which come from the kidneys. With very overweight women amenorrhoea is generally due to damp and phlegm, and to the fat in the membranes causing a blockage. There will be other manifestations of blockage due to damp and phlegm, for instance congestion and oppression in the chest, nausea, and abundant vaginal discharges which are often white. There is a general lack of transportation and transformation leading to oedema or a buildup of liquids internally. Treatment should focus on expelling the damp and resolving the blockages to re-establish healthy circulation and communication.

Invasion of heat in the blood chamber

We will now look at chapter 22 of the Jingui yaolüe. The title of this book, Jingui yaolüe, is often translated as Essential Prescriptions of the Golden Coffer or Essentials from the Golden Cabinet. The same author also wrote the Shanghanlun. His name was Zhong Ji, but he is better known as Zhang Zhongjing, and he lived in the second half of the 2nd century and the beginning of the 3rd century CE. There are three chapters in the Jingui yaolüe devoted to women's diseases, generally taken as chapters 20, 21 and 22, referring to pregnant women, postpartum conditions and miscellaneous gynaecological diseases respectively.

Chapter 22, on miscellaneous gynaecological

diseases, details four types of injury all resulting in heat entering the blood chamber and causing disturbance to menstruation and the woman's behaviour. The four injuries have the same consequence but all have different symptoms and treatment:

> 'Injury due to the wind in women: after six or seven days, the patient has cold chills and fever with timely onset of the crisis and menstruation ceases. This is a case of invasion of heat in the blood chamber (*re ru xue shi* 熱入血室). The knots (*jie* 結) made by the blood are the cause of this timely onset [of cold and heat] resembling intermittent fevers. The lesser bupleurum decoction (*xiao chai hu tang* 小柴胡湯) treats it.
>
> Injury due to the cold with excess of fever in women: when menstruation arrives the patient is clear [in her mind] during the day, but has delirium and insanity at night. It is like when someone has hallucinations of demons. This is a case of invasion of heat in the blood chamber. To treat take care not to offend the stomach *qi* or the two upper heaters. It will heal by itself.
>
> Injury due to the cold with excess of fever and sensitivity to the cold in women: seven to eight days after the beginning of her menstruation, the fever disappears, the pulse becomes slow, the body is cool (cold) and she has fullness (*man*

滿) in the chest and the ribs area, similar to the knots in the chest (*jie xiong* 結胸), and she has delirium. This is a case of invasion of heat in the blood chamber. Needle on *qi men* (Liver 14), to let out the fullness (*shi* 實).

Yang ming diseases with bleeding from the lower [orifices] and delirium, and with sweat coming out at the head: this is a case of invasion of heat in the blood chamber. Needle on *qi men* (Liver 14) to disperse the (*yang ming*) fullness (*shi* 實). When the sweat comes out on the whole body, it is a sign of recovery.'

The same expression keeps repeating itself here: 'This is a case of invasion of heat in the blood chamber (*re ru xue shi* 熱入血室)'. The 'blood chamber' (*xue shi* 血室) can be interpreted in three different ways, which are really the same. It can be the liver, the *chong mai* or the uterus. Even if we choose one interpretation rather than another it is just a question of point of view not of meaning since the functions of all three are the same. If we take 'blood chamber' as the liver, it means the liver is responsible for retaining and releasing the blood and thus regulating the flow of blood to and within the uterus. If we take it as referring to the *chong mai* we include all the movement of the *zang* and *fu* in making the blood, and the *qi* regulating the movement of the blood. Finally, if it is the uterus it is the place where all these functions are expressed through the blood arriving, resting and leaving.

The approach in the Jingui yaolüe is different from that found in the Shanghanlun. The Shanghanlun concentrates on external pathogenic agents invading stage by stage. In the Jingui yaolüe the presentation is made by categories of disease, for example, everything which is relevant to the blockage or disturbance of the lung. It is interesting to compare the first paragraph from the Jingui yaolüe with a passage from the Shanghanlun:

> 'Injury due to the wind in women: after six or seven days the patient has cold chills and fever with timely onset of the crisis and menstruation ceases. This is a case of invasion of heat in the blood chamber. The knots made by the blood are the cause of this timely onset [of cold and heat] resembling intermittent fevers. The lesser bupleurum decoction (*xiao chai hu tang*) treats it.' (Jingui yaolüe chapter 22, paragraph 1)

> 'The woman has an injury by the wind (*zhong feng* 中風) and after seven or eight days she has periodic chills and fever [in alternation], and the menstruation stops. This means that the heat has entered the blood chamber. There will be knots in the blood and this is the reason why there are intermittent fevers. Lesser bupleurum decoction (*xiao chai hu tang*) governs.' (Shanghanlun paragraph 144 or 150)

This is an injury from an attack by external perverse wind, which takes advantage of a weakness in the woman and the circulation in her lower abdomen to penetrate the blood chamber. The woman is struck by the pathogen when she is vulnerable and weak at the time of menstruation, or at the end of menstruation when she is in a state of emptiness of blood and unrest in the *qi*. When she finishes menstruation, after six or seven days she starts to show symptoms of chills and fever. The 'timely onset' of the crisis means that the chills and fever are a regular occurrence, they do not come randomly. Therefore, the wind and heat come from the outside first, or as a result of the attack inside of the body.

It is very easy to have wind and heat due to wind at the end of menstruation when there is a weakness and emptiness of blood. The wind allows the heat to develop inside the body, and the heat, pushed by the wind, enters the blood of the uterus and menstruation. This is the reason for the regular appearance of the fever. Because of the wind there may be a blockage of the liver and gallbladder, and the heat in the blood may prevent good circulation of the blood. There may be clots of blood in the uterus, which are an expression of the heat in the blood chamber. The remedy given for this is *xiao chai hu tang*, lesser bupleurum decoction (*xiao chai hu tang* 小柴胡湯).

The second example given in the Jingue yaolüe is injury due to cold with excessive fever:

'Injury due to the cold with excess of fever in women: when menstruation arrives the patient is clear [in her mind] during the day, but has delirium and insanity at night. It is like when someone has hallucinations of demons. This is a case of invasion of heat in the blood chamber. To treat take care not to offend the stomach *qi* or the two upper heaters. It will heal by itself.'

This is similar to another Shanghanlun paragraph: 'The woman has an injury by the cold (*shang han* 傷寒) with fever when the menstruation arrives, she is clear headed during the day and speaks deliriously in the evening as if hallucinating ghosts. This means that the heat has entered the blood chamber. But if there is no assault on the stomach *qi* or on the two upper burners, she will recover spontaneously.' (Shanghanlun paragraph 145 or 150)

In this case the woman receives an external attack by perverse *qi* at the time of her menstruation. The original pathogen is the cold, but it makes a blockage and generates heat by transformation. This is the heat which penetrates the blood chamber. Or it is the cold which causes the blockage in the lower abdomen which generates the heat that penetrates the blood chamber. That is very typical of the way Zhang Zhongjing works things out in his mind. The woman is insane during the night, but during the day she is normal and clear.

If the woman is clear headed during the day and only confused in the night time, it is not a case of heat in the stomach. In both the Shanghanlun and the Jingue yaolüe we have to eliminate the wrong diagnosis. It is not heat in the stomach because if it were, the woman would be insane all the time. With heat in the stomach she would be even more agitated during the day than during the night. This is a sign that the cause of the delirium is not located in the upper or middle heater. It leads us to the lower heater and this is something which is at the level of the blood, and heat in the blood in the lower heater.

In such a situation you have to be sure not to treat the upper and middle heaters since that would provoke further symptoms and weaken the women even more. No purging treatments should be given for the middle heater since they would be useless therapeutically and would damage her, increasing her delirium. This is because when menstruation stops her delirious speech will also stop since the heat will have been eliminated with the blood. You just have to wait for that time. If you do nothing to hinder the normal descent of the blood the woman will recover by herself. You can assist the process with the right diagnosis and treatment, for instance with some variation of the lesser bupleurum decoction. But you must avoid anything which increases the rising up or springing out movements of *qi*, and you must not induce sweating or vomiting because these will weaken the *qi* which helps the blood come out through the uterus. With acupuncture you can use a point such as Liver 14 to sustain the correct movement of *qi*, or Kidney 8, which is the *xi* cleft point of the *yin qiao mai*. Heart Master 4 is the *xi* cleft point of the *xin zhu* meridian (or *jue yin* of the hand), and will help clear the heat from the blood.

The third paragraph from the Jingui Yaolüe says:

'Injury due to the cold with excess of fever and sensitivity to the cold in women: seven to eight days after the beginning of her menstruation, the fever disappears, the pulse becomes slow, the body is cool (cold) and she has fullness (*man* 滿) in the chest and the ribs area, similar to the knots in the chest (*jie xiong* 結胸), and she has delirium. This is a case of invasion of heat in the blood chamber. Needle on *qi men* (Liver 14), to let out the fullness (*shi* 實).'

This is comparable to paragraph 143 (or 148) from the Shanghanlun:

'The woman has an injury by the wind and she has cold chills and fever [in alternation] and the menstruation arrives. If after seven or eight days the fever has ceased and the pulse is slow, her whole body is cold, she is congested in the chest and under the ribs, like in chest knots, and she speaks deliriously. This means that the heat has entered the blood chamber. One should needle *qi men* (Liver 14) in order to treat the fullness.'

During menstruation the sea of blood and the chamber of blood will empty, so it is at that time the woman is open to receive an injury by the wind. This is the same thing as we saw in the first paragraphs where the pathogenic factor entered the woman easily and created heat in the liver, and via the liver into the chamber of blood, the uterus or *chong mai*, whatever the chamber of blood is exactly. The meridians of the liver and gallbladder are infiltrated by the inner wind and produce symptoms which are half physical and half mental. To begin with the woman will have alternating chills and fever which are symptoms linked to the *biao* (表), the exterior. This reaction is easily connected with the gallbladder meridian. After these the fever ceases, the pulse is slow and the body is cool. This means that the symptoms are no longer in the exterior but have penetrated into the interior (*li* 裡). The perverse is now in the blood blocking the circulation and this is why there is a slowness in the pulse.

Once the pathogenic factor is in the liver, the blood and the blood chamber, the liver cannot function properly so there is congestion in the ribs and chest. This is similar to what is called 'knots in the chest', but it is not exactly the same thing because that is a symptom related to the *tai yang* amongst other things. These knots come as a result of the perverse *qi* which has penetrated the depths of the body. In the Shanghanlun chest knots are normally related to symptoms in the exterior, the *biao*. However, the feeling or sensation is the same, and the woman will feel the same sort of congestion.

Because the heat which enters the blood of the lower heater may be spread to the heart by the liver, there is a disturbance in the heart and mind, resulting in the delirium. The problem is really in the liver and the blood of the liver, so treatment must try to soften the liver and establish better circulation of the blood and all the connections of the blood. The point Liver 14 is used to restore local circulation, and free the liver from pathogenic fullness and obstruction. It is also the *mu* point of the liver, which is good for any kind of stagnation or stasis, and specifically when there is a relationship with heat. Other points such as Triple Heater 5 and Gallbladder 41 help improve the circulation.

The fourth paragraph of the Jingue yaolüe is as follows:

> '*Yang ming* (陽 明) diseases with bleeding from the lower [orifices] and delirium, and with sweat coming out at the head: this is a case of invasion of heat in the blood chamber. Needle on *qi men* (Liver 14) to disperse the (*yang ming*) fullness (*shi* 實). When the sweat comes out on the whole body, it is a sign of recovery.'

This is the descent of the blood from the vagina with a lot of delirium. This is very similar to paragraph 216 (or 221 in other editions) of the Shanghanlun:

> '*Yang ming* disease with descending of blood and delirious speech: this means that the heat has

entered the blood chamber. If the sweat comes out only from the head, one should needle *qi men* (Liver 14) in order to disperse the fullness. When the sweat is all around the body it is a sign of recovering.'

In this situation the perverse heat follows the *yang ming* meridian, and creates pressure on the blood in the lower abdomen, mainly in the chamber of blood. Therefore the symptoms develop in the uterus and *chong mai* and in the circulation of the menstrual blood. Here the heat in the blood in the lower abdomen and the *yang ming* cause a counter current in the *chong mai* because of the solidarity between the *chong mai* and the *yang ming* of the stomach. If there is heat in the blood in the lower abdomen there will also be a counter current in the liver and its meridian. There is not only the pressure exerted by the heat on the blood at the level of the lower orifices, but also heat in the blood rising up via the counter current of the liver. Hence the delirium.

The heat and counter current in the liver meridian and *chong mai* will continue and prevent the descending movement of the *qi* and its normal spreading out. The heat pushing upwards disturbs the correct movement of the *yang qi* in such a way that sweating occurs only at the head. This is the reason why it is a sign of recovery when the sweating is all over the body because it is a sign that the *qi* has recovered its normal circulation throughout the whole body. By means of the sweat the remaining heat can be eliminated. Needling Liver 14 disperses the fullness of heat in the liver meridian, and calms the wind agitation, thus allowing the heat in the blood and uterus to be dispersed. When the correct circulation of the *yang qi* of all the meridians has been restored then there will be sweat throughout the whole body, and recovery is on its way.

These four paragraphs of the Jingue yaolüe and the Shanghanlun are interesting because of the discussion of the entrance of heat into the blood chamber. This is something very important in gynaecology as it is found in ancient texts.

Invasion by cold

In paragraph 8 of the same chapter 22 of the Jingue yaolüe there is another passage which is significant for gynaecology. Both cold in the blood and cold in the uterus are described, and three main causes in disturbance to menstruation are discussed. In this section a differentiation is made according to the three levels of the body:

> 'Women's disease with emptiness (*xu* 虛) or accumulation of cold, and knotting of the *qi* (*jie qi* 結氣), can cause the menstruation to stop for up to one year. The cold in the blood causes accumulation and knots, the cervix of the uterus is injured by the cold, and circulation in the

meridians and connective pathways (*jing luo* 經絡) is blocked, as if frozen.

In the upper part there is vomiting of saliva and liquids and spitting. If it lasts a long time there will be abscesses in the lung and her whole body will become emaciated. In the centre the cold either causes pain on both sides of the navel or the pain is located on both sides of the ribs with a dragging pain radiating towards the *zang* (the liver). Or the knots give rise to heat in the centre with pain at *guan yuan*, Ren 4. The pulse is rapid. There are no sores, but the skin is scaly. This may also affect male patients.

In the lower part, there is continuous bleeding after the normal end of menstruation. There is irregular menstruation with dragging pain toward the uterus and vagina. They may also be either sensitivity to the cold in the lower abdomen, or pain radiating towards the lumbar region and the spine, descending toward the street of *qi* (*qi jie* 氣街, one of the names of Stomach 30) where it seems to root. Painful pressure is felt at the thoroughfare of *qi* (*qi chong* 氣衝, the other of the two names of Stomach 30). The knees and legs are painful and ill at ease. The woman has sudden mental confusion with dizziness, vertigo and blurred vision, as someone who is mad. The woman can feel unhappy and sad, grieving with a lot of anger. All these symptoms are dependent on gynaecological diseases and are not due to spirits and ghosts. If it lasts a long time the woman becomes emaciated, the pulses are empty and the sensitivity to the cold is great.'

The pain starts first on both sides of the navel, or alternatively it starts in the rib area and radiates towards the *zang*, which in this context almost certainly means the liver. But there is another possibility which is that the cold makes a blockage which evolves into knots and inner heat. Heat in the centre ends with a pain located at the level of *guan yuan* (關元), which is Ren 4.

The passage gives the example of cold in the blood leading to accumulation, knots and blockage, which is called cold at the level of the kidneys. The kidneys are the water *qi* and if they are cold they are unable to balance water and fire, *yin* and *yang*, and therefore are unable to support the dynamism and prosperity of the wood movement of the liver. The blood cannot circulate so you get stasis, knots, and cold in the areas where the blood circulates.

First there will be an effect in the upper part of the body. This will be mainly as a consequence of the cold of the stomach and lung, with the formation of phlegm and pathological body fluids, hence the spitting and vomiting of liquids. If the cold settles in this area and is not expelled or warmed up there will be a blockage of the *qi*. But in this case, if there is still enough *yang* or defensive *qi* there will be a struggle between the perverse *qi* (*xie qi* 邪氣) and the correct *qi* (*zheng qi* 正氣) and there will be the reaction to the blockage of *qi* by the cold, generating inner heat. This heat has an effect on the phlegm which in turn will provoke abscesses in the lung. Therefore there is a perverse fullness in the upper part of the body. But at this stage of the process it is still possible to disperse and clarify the heat, not forgetting that there is an emptiness of the kidneys. Cold is present there. This is the reason treatment has to warm up and nourish the emptiness of the kidneys. Cold in the kidneys and blockage in the upper part are reasons for bad circulation of nutrition and subsequent loss of weight.

In the centre or middle heater, if there is a blockage of liver *qi* the effects will also be felt in the spleen and stomach. This is why the pain is around the navel and the radiation of the pain is towards the liver. The pain is due to the presence of the cold but there may be reactive heat due to the blockage of the *qi*, in which case the pain will be under the navel. This is because the inner heat is in the blood of the lower abdomen. The pain is in the lower abdomen because the inner heat, due to the cold and the blockage, has entered in the blood of the uterus. It happens because the liver, responsible for the blood of the uterus, is injured, blocked and has reactive heat.

Heat in the lower abdomen produces a reaction in the skin which is linked to the *tai yang* quality or level of *qi*, and to the defensive *qi*, *wei qi*. The *qi* of the lower abdomen normally circulates in the superficial layers of the body, so this is why there may be an effect visible on the skin. If there is heat present it has an effect on the nourishment of the skin and the heat dries up the skin and provokes scaliness. But there are no actual sores since there is no damp heat at the skin, and there will not be sores around the mouth. The heat explains the rapid pulse. This is something which occurs in a man as well as a woman.

In the lower part of the body the cold injures the circulation and causes blood stasis and blockage of the *qi*. There is obstruction of the liver resulting in irregular menstruation and pain. There is not only the first effect of the cold but also the possibility of reactive heat, so there is a violent counter current which arises from the area of Stomach 30, *qi chong*, the thoroughfare of *qi*. This is the emerging point of the *chong mai*. The pain is in the lower area of the body or the abdomen, but the patient has the feeling that the root of the pain is coming from Stomach 30.

There is a double association of the *chong mai* with the *yang ming* and *shao yin* of the foot, that is the stomach and kidney meridians. It is through the association of the *chong mai* and the kidney meridian that there may be weakness and pain in the knees and legs. The cold in the blood disturbs the functioning of the *zang* and may lead to psychological disorder because of the lack of clear *yang* rising up to nourish the heart and the spirits of the heart, or from a lack of clear essences in the blood to nourish the liver and the *hun*. Whenever there is a disturbance by cold there is a lack of mental clarity involving heart and liver. A woman with a gynaecological problem such as bleeding or vaginal discharge may become weaker and weaker with the pulses presenting a weak and empty aspect, and she will feel cold or very sensitive to the cold. This explains the last sentence of the passage: 'If it lasts a long time the patient will lose weight, the pulses will be empty and there will be great sensitivity to the cold.'

This is a long quotation but it is a very good one because it contains many things. The clinical observation is excellent and accurate, and all the internal movements are explained.

Paragraph 6 in the same chapter 22 mentions a symptom called *zang zao* (藏 躁). *Zao* (躁) means agitation:

> 'The woman has an agitation in the *zang* (*zang zao* 藏 躁). She is easily sad with a desire to cry. It is as if she was under supernatural or magical influences (*shen ling* 神 靈). She stretches and yawns frequently. The decoction of licorice, wheat and jujube (*gan mai da zao tang* 甘 麥 大 棗 湯) masters this.'

This is a situation in which the woman appears to be suffering under some magical influence. She stretches and yawns frequently. The treatment is to give *gan mai da zao tang* which contains liquorice, wheat and jujube. This woman has anxieties, worries, oppression and despondency, and is unable to free herself from these feelings. This is a case of blockage or exhaustion of the *yin* so there will be dryness of the blood. The body fluids, particularly the *jin* (津) liquids, will also be injured and diminished. The weakness of the *yin* and the essences which are the foundation and nourishment of the *zang*, leads to agitation disturbing the mind deeply, so the woman will continuously change from tears to laughter, elation to sadness (*xi bei* 喜悲), without reason, as if someone had commanded these fluctuations by magic. She is not in possession of herself, and just follows something external. In this situation the lack of essences cannot ensure the presence of the spirits which guarantee her self-possession and the reality of herself.

If all the *zang* are disturbed by the lack of essences there may be a surging of one emotion or another, depending on the disorder. The agitation is also in the *zang*. '*Zang*' in this context represents the heart because it is the heart which is responsible for all the emotions, receiving the movements of the five *zang* which make the emotional life and the calm, peacefulness of the mind. However, if the supply of essences is not good or rich enough the spirits cannot manifest their presence because of the agitation which exists in the heart.

Occasionally some commentaries say that the *zang* referred to here is the lung. This is because the sadness comes first, so it is understood as a blockage of the *qi* of the chest due to that sadness. The blockage of the movement of the lung *qi* creates the agitation in the upper heater leading to mental disturbance characterised by a tendency to sadness (*xi bei* 喜 悲). For many other commentators the *zang* is the uterus, the place where essences are kept. Therefore this is an agitation in the uterus and the blood causing heat in the blood chamber and leading to delirium or delirious speech. In this case there is the link with what in western terminology we call 'hysteria'. Of course the word hysteria itself derives from the ancient Greek for womb.

It is also easy to say that there is an emptiness and a dryness of blood, and an emptiness of the liver *yin*. The liquids are involved as well, so there is a diminishing of the bodily liquids, mainly perceptible in the lung. Between the liver and the lung, and the blood and the liquids, both become damaged and dry up. The explanation of the fluctuating emotions, the sadness and the tears, and the stretching of the body to try to unblock the circulation of *qi* is that these things are very often characteristics of an obstruction of the liver. There are usually symptoms of agitation and uneasiness from the heart, heat, dryness or insomnia, as well as symptoms such as constipation coming from the lack of the *jin* (津) liquids in the intestines, because the large intestine is related to the lung.

If the *zang* referred to is the heart we can understand how all the irregularities may arise because the heart is open to all the different *qi* which themselves come erratically from the other *zang* deprived of essences and blood. It could also be an emptiness of the blood of the uterus, for instance due to wind and heat in the uterus, which causes symptoms in the liver and heart.

This is nearly the same pattern. Certainly the kidneys are involved in the fundamental decreasing of the *yin*, and yawning is often associated with the kidneys. Sometimes stretching is also related to the kidneys because it indicates the body trying to establish a better communication and harmony between *yin* and *yang*.

Gan mai da zao tang, the treatment which is suggested, is interesting because it tries to nourish the heart and the spleen in order to relax tension and blockage in the liver. This is the reason the wheat is included because wheat is the grain specially appropriate for the liver. It harmonizes liver *qi* and is also very good for nourishing the heart. In this formula the wheat (*mai* 麥) takes the position of master or sovereign herb (*jun* 君). In position of minister or helper herbs there are licorice (*gan cao* 甘草) and jujube (*da zao* 大棗), because both are able to nourish the *yin*, especially the *yin* of the heart and the spleen, and these two herbs harmonize the centre and thus relax tension. The three herbs together make a remedy which is sweet and well balanced (*gan ping* 甘平). The sweet taste is able to tonify and nourish the emptiness of the *yin* in the heart and spleen, but the sweet taste is also used to relax the tension and so to calm the liver, the centre and all the internal agitation.

As it says in Suwen chapter 22, when there is tension in the liver you have to eat sweet to relax.

There are a lot of possibilities with acupuncture treatment too. A point such as Du 26 is good because it is a place of exchange between the *du* and *ren mai* and the *yin* and the *yang*. It is good as a revival point in case of great hysteria for example. To help re-establish the clear *yang* in the heart, the upper orifices and the brain it can be used with Du 20. Heart Master 6 and Heart 7 work on the blockage in the chest and will calm the counter current due to the heat and lack of *yin*. Heart 7 calms the spirits and the mind. Liver 3 frees the circulation of the liver, eliminates obstruction there and calms the wind.

For someone who is always laughing and crying you could add points such as Heart Master 5, which is the right point for this. It can be used with a point such as Small Intestine 3. If there is a counter current of *qi* with a blockage and pressure in the chest, it is better to use points such as Ren 17 or even Stomach 40, which is also useful when there is the disturbance of the body liquids and phlegm. In case of mental disturbance it is possible to needle Bladder 15 to tonify the deficiency of nutrition in the heart. Bladder 47, *hun men* (魂門), the point at the same level as the *shu* (輸) point of the liver, is also helpful for mental disorder. But of course with all these treatments you have to remember to look at the causes and to nourish and sustain.

INDEX

INDEX

amenorrhoea 22, 41, 91, 92, 93, 95-107
Analects 4
anger 15, 35, 78, 79, 85, 93, 98, 119
ancestral qi 103
anterior heaven 27, 35, 47, 49
Art of the Heart 7

bao luo 18-25, 44
bao mai 18, 21, 43
bao zhong 11, 19-21, 43, 47
bladder 69, 33
Bladder 15 89, 127
Bladder 17 83, 97
Bladder 18 89, 97
Bladder 20 81, 90, 97
Bladder 23 76, 89, 90
Bladder 25 97
Bladder 31 81
Bladder 32 99
Bladder 33 83
Bladder 47 126
Bladder 62 17
blood chamber 108, 109, 110, 114, 124
blood stasis 82, 97-99
bones 23, 58, 60, 61, 66, 74, 75, 101
Book of Rites 6, 7, 62,
Book of Change 56
brain 23, 28
breasts 79, 80

Chunqiu zuozhuan 3
cold 8, 75, 98, 118
conception 26, 50, 74, 82, 92
Confucius 4
constipation 88, 98, 125

dai mai 52-53, 76
damp 38, 53, 72, 73, 75, 80-81, 91, 93, 99, 106-107

delirium   115
depression   89, 90
diarrhoea   32, 40, 76
dizziness   81, 87, 95, 101, 119
dream   80, 91
dryness   88, 125
du mai   19, 30, 37, 50-52
Du 4   52, 76, 81, 90, 91
Du 20   83, 87, 126
Du 26   126

earth   3, 6, 23, 59, 63, 70, 71
embryo   1, 2, 29, 50, 68, 74, 78, 82
emotion   4, 6, 7, 33, 44, 84, 97, 106, 124
eyes   94, 95

fertility   27, 48, 49, 50, 52, 54-71
fever   77, 88, 104, 105, 107, 110-115
fire   26, 28, 30, 31, 51, 59, 85
four limbs   92, 94
four seasons   8, 56
Furen daquanliangfang   100

gallbladder 23, 24, 25, 34, 52, 69
gallbladder meridian   53, 114, 115
Gallbladder 26   52, 76
Gallbladder 41   116
gan mai du zao tang   123, 125
genitals   25, 30, 33, 36
ghosts   119
Guanzi   2

haemorrhage   30, 33, 40, 44, 93
hair   11, 12-13, 37, 58, 60, 61, 66, 69, 67, 71, 103
Heart 7   89, 126
heart master meridian   20
Heart Master 4   113
Heart Master 6   80, 97, 99, 126
Heart Master 5   127

Heart Master 7   89
heat   30, 44, 46, 104, 107-118
heaven   1, 2, 6, 62
hot flushes   88, 104
Huainanzi   8
Huangdi   54-55
hun   87
hysteria   124

infertility   1, 72-83
insanity   108, 111
insomnia   17, 87, 88, 91, 105, 125

jealousy   15, 35, 78, 93
jing shen   20, 30, 61, 62
Jingui yaolüe   1, 107, 109, 110, 113, 116, 117, 118
jin ye, body fluids   38, 125
jue yin   20, 43

kidney *qi*   5, 58, 59, 60, 61, 64
kidney meridian 22, 39, 49, 122
Kidney 3   76, 83, 89
Kidney 6   17, 99
Kidney 8   113
knees   77, 88, 101, 119, 122

lactation   27, 34, 40, 46, 48
Large Int 4   80, 99
Lingshu chapter 10   20
Lingshu chapter 13   36
Lingshu chapter 17   16
Lingshu chapter 33   35
Lingshu chapter 65   10-12, 19, 48
liver fire   31, 89
liver meridian   33, 37, 46, 49, 79, 80, 94, 114, 117
liver tendino-muscular   36
Liver 3   80, 81, 126
Liver 8   98
Liver 14   52, 108, 113, 114, 115, 117
lung meridian   21
Lunyu   4

madness   119
marrow   23, 28, 60, 74, 75, 76, 101
menopause   1, 71, 83-91
menstruation   1, 13, 30, 33, 35, 38, 40, 64, 65, 75, 76, 91
ming men   20, 51, 52, 75, 90
miscarriage   68, 73, 83, 86, 96
moon   8-9
muscles   16, 17, 33, 36, 58, 66, 71, 86

Nanjing difficult issue 27   39
Nanjing difficult issue 29   17, 48
Nanjing difficult issue 36   20, 22
Nanjing difficult issue 39   20, 22
night fever   104

obsession   15, 91, 97
oppression   79, 90, 97, 99, 106, 123
origin   27, 28
ovaries   37

palpitations   77, 81, 88, 91, 97, 102, 103, 105
phlegm   72, 80-81, 91, 93, 99, 106-107, 120
posterior heaven   27, 38, 39, 47, 68
pregnancy   2, 22, 27, 34, 39, 49, 68, 74, 83

Qi Bo   54, 55
qi heng zhi fu, extraordinary fu   23, 24
qiao mai   15-17

Ren 2   37
Ren 3   40, 81, 98
Ren 4   49, 81, 90, 97, 119, 120
Ren 5   81
Ren 6   81, 90, 91
Ren 8   81

sadness   7, 44, 123, 124, 125
sea of blood   35, 39, 40, 48, 70, 93, 101, 114
sea of meridians   11, 48
sea of qi   36, 90, 103
sexual desire   5, 29, 30

Shanghanlun   107, 109, 110, 115, 118
shao yang   56
shao yin   56, 122
skin   11, 12, 13, 68, 69, 70, 82, 89, 103, 119, 121
Small Int 3   126
sperm   2, 25, 35, 56
spirits   8, 19, 89, 122, 124
spleen meridian   43, 49
Spleen 6   80, 81, 83, 89, 97, 99
Spleen 8   98
Spleen 10   89, 97
stomach meridian   34, 46
Stomach 25   97
Stomach 28   81
Stomach 29   80, 81, 90
Stomach 30   98, 119, 122
Stomach 36   97, 98
Stomach 40   127
Suwen chapter 1   1, 13, 28, 48, 54-72, 73, 83, 86
Suwen chapter 5   56, 67
Suwen chapter 7   91
Suwen chapter 11   23, 25
Suwen chapter 21   45
Suwen chapter 22   126
Suwen chapter 26   8
Suwen chapter 33   21, 22, 43
Suwen chapter 40   92, 104
Suwen chapter 44   39, 40
Suwen chapter 47   22
Suwen chapter 60   39, 48, 51
sweating   79, 113, 116, 117

tai yang   56, 115, 121
Tang dynasty   50
tai yin   56
teeth   58, 60, 61, 65, 66
tian gui, fertility   61-65
thirst   88
tinnitus   75, 87, 101
Triple Heater 5   116

vaginal discharge 53, 76, 81, 105, 119, 122
vaginal mucus 41
vertigo 77, 87, 88, 95, 119
vomiting 81, 113, 118, 120

Wanshinüke 105
Wan Quan 105
Wang Bing 50
wei qi, defensive qi 8, 29, 121
wind 110, 114, 117
wisdom teeth 65
worry 78, 91, 96, 97, 102

xiao chai hu tang 108, 110
xin bao 18-25
xin bao luo 18, 20
xin zhu 41, 43
xing, nature 6
xue ku, dryness of the blood 96-97
Xunzi 5, 6

yang ming 39, 40, 47, 48, 58, 68, 116, 117
yawning 123, 125
Ye Gui 102
Yeshinüke zhengzhi 107
Yixue zhengzhuan 100
yuan qi, original *qi* 20
Yu Tuan 100

zao, agitation 123
Zhang jiebin 40, 104
Zhang Zhongjing 107, 112
zhen, authentic 27
zheng qi, correct *qi* 120
Zhong Ji 107
Zhuangqingzhunüke 78, 80
zong jin, ancestral muscle 35, 36
zong qi, ancestral *qi* 35, 103